Modern Carbon Point-based Impedimetric G4 Sensors for Microorganisms Identification

Y. Narayan

Contents

Chapter 1

Introduction

1. Introduction

Bacterial infection is one of the biggest threats to mankind, and the infectious diseases associated with it have an invincible catastrophe, affecting millions of lives annually [1,2]. In the last few decades, a significant rise in infectious diseases due to antibiotic resistance bacteria has become prominent [3–5]. This sharp increase in antibiotic-resistant/multi-drug resistant (MDR) bacteria is alarming as approximately 8-9 million mortality cases have already been reported [6–10]. With this pace, the expected death toll may surge beyond 10 million cases globally, with an additional economic burden of 100.2 trillion dollars by 2050 [10–12]. The rapid emergence of MDR is due to the use and misuse of antibiotics during blind treatment and healthcare mismanagement with a life-threatening outcome. MDR existence could be due to different types of mutations such as changes at the antibiotic target site, cell wall permeability, or in the carrier [13,14].

MDR bacteria virulence causing factors are mainly available on the cell wall, and the pathogenicity can be identified by studying the cell wall components [15,16]. Majorly, two classes of bacteria have been categorized on the basis of cell wall configuration and was used in Gram staining technique for differentiating into Gram-positive and Gram-negative bacteria (Fig. 1.1). The cell wall composition of Gram-positive bacteria constitutes a thick peptidoglycan membrane having two important alternating sugar residues of β-(1,4) linked N-acetylglucosamine (NAG) and N-acetylmuramic acid (NAM). The peptidoglycan layer is followed by a layer of polymeric teichoic acid and cytoplasmic membrane. Gram-negative bacteria are composed of thin peptidoglycan layers in between the outer lipopolysaccharide (LPS) membrane and inner cytoplasmic membrane. The lipopolysaccharide is a toxic layer that results in the generation of an immune response. It consists of lipid A, core polysaccharide, O & H antigen and may cause septic shock [17,18].

In general, there are significant differences in the composition of bacterial cell wall. The several pathogenic bacteria have unique cell wall arrangements in terms of membrane phospholipid, protein ratio, and the net charges available on the cell surface [19,20]. Therefore, it is reasonable to say that the cell walls are bacteria fingerprints that can effectively identify different bacteria.

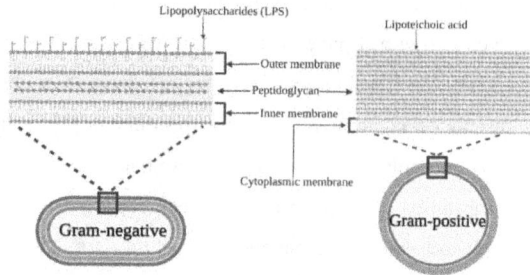

Fig.1.1 Gram-negative (rod shaped E. coli as a model organism) and Gram-positive (spherical S. aureus as a model organism) bacterial cell composition analysis

The pathogenic bacteria having MDR property comes under a popular acronym as "ESKAPE" (*Enterococcus faecium, Staphylococcus aureus, Klebsiella pneumoniae, Acinetobacter baumannii, Pseudomonas aeruginosa*, and *Enterobacter species*) microorganisms [21,22]. As the acronym suggests, the MDR bacteria tend to prevent themselves from the several antibiotics due to which the lethality increases exponentially [23,24]. Therefore, essential steps should be taken to curb the spike in MDR bacteria, such as maintain good hygiene, pace up the synthesis of new antibiotics, antibiotics management while treating patients, and rapid, efficient, and real-time monitoring of pathogenic bacteria [25–27].

The advent of MDR bacteria can also be significantly controlled by rapid and precise surveillance [28]. The exact screening may also help in identifying the new infections and resistance developed in pathogenic bacteria and aid in healthcare management [29]. Moreover, the sensitive and selective detection of MDR bacteria at low cost and short turn-around time is required to curb the possible outbreak.

1.1 Bacterial detection techniques

The traditional methods for bacteria detection have been summarized in Fig. 1.2. The gold standard assay *viz*; cell culture assay, molecular diagnostics, and immunoassay have been described in the following sections.

2

1.1.1 Cell culture assay (Gold standard)

Considered the 'gold-standard assay', bacterial culturing is one of the most reliable and common bacterial identification methods in microbiology [30–32]. The culturing assay is carried out using culture media having all the nutrients essential for the growth and multiplication of bacteria at standard conditions such as pH, temperature, and ionic conditions [33,34]. The culture media could be liquid or solid and is called liquid broth or solid agar media, respectively. These two media variants come under a commercial name as Luria Bertani (LB) media (broth/agar). The LB media could be deployed to identify Gram-positive and Gram-negative bacteria [35–38].

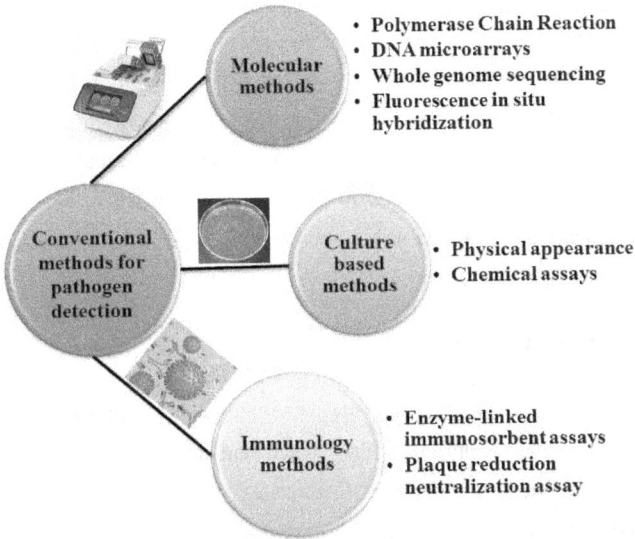

Fig. 1.2 Conventional diagnostic assays for the detection of pathogenic bacteria

The major drawback of cell culturing assay is the time required for obtaining the result from the time of sample collection. The cell culture assay requires at least 72 hours to confirm if the infection was caused due to specific bacteria present in a clinical sample [39,40].

3

1.1.2 Matrix-assisted laser desorption/ionization-time of flight mass spectrometry (MALDI-TOF MS)

Rapid diagnosis is one of the fundamental requirements to provide necessary treatment to ailing patients and refrain from the emergence and spread of MDR bacteria. MALDI-TOF MS has influenced pathogen detection in terms of speed and accuracy [41,42]. The application of MALDI-TOF MS in bacterial detection relies on identifying ribosomal proteins as major biomolecules of interest. Each bacterium has its unique protein with characteristic mass and forms the basis of detection of MALDI-TOF MS. These proteins of different mass provide a "fingerprint" for different bacteria and can be stored in the repository to identify the genus and species. Currently, MS uses bacterial culture to identify microbes grown on selective media but possesses certain limitations [43]. MALDI-TOF MS cannot identify taxonomically related bacteria such as differentiating between highly pathogenic *Shigella* species from commensal *E. coli* variant and *Streptococcus pneumoniae* from commensal streptococci. The drawbacks extend to the culture requirement wherein the time requirement can rise to 24 hours or more. Also, the expensive and bulkier instrumentation and high power consumption are other disadvantages associated with MALDI-TOF MS [44,45].

1.1.3 In-situ hybridization

The molecular diagnostic techniques depend on specific gene sequences or genomic markers comprising the nucleic acid sequences. These genomic markers can also be defined as molecular "fingerprints" to characterize pathogenic bacteria and provide information on their genus, species, and viability. The molecular diagnosis of pathogenic bacteria depends on amplifying specific gene sequences or sequencing the target gene, such as ribosomal genes[46,47].

In this method, the single or double-stranded short oligonucleotide probes tagged with fluorescent dyes (Cy3/ FITC) are deployed for detecting the target gene. The complementary nature of the probes helps in binding with the target gene. This probe-target hybridization is confirmed by the fluorescence emitted by the bounded probe when excited with the light source of a specific wavelength. This is called fluorescence in-situ hybridization (FISH). Peptide nucleic acid oligomers-based FISH (PNA-FISH) was used for the identification of Gram-positive and Gram-negative bacteria in the blood sample [48]. The disadvantages associated with this technique include sensitivity, selectivity, and applicability to a smaller range of bacterial pathogens [49].

1.1.4 Polymerase Chain Reaction (PCR)

The amplification of the gene of interest using PCR is the backbone of molecular diagnostic techniques. This technique has been used immensely to provide faster and sensitive results. In general, PCR includes amplifying genes with the help of a specifically designed primer to amplify the gene of a certain nucleic acid sequence (Fig. 1.3). The program should be set for a fixed number of cycles to amplify the target DNA sequence [50,51]. Different strategies exist to amplify the gene of interest available in different pathogenic bacteria [52–54]. On a similar note, real-time PCR (RT-PCR) is used to measure the fluorescence signal emitted from the primers labeled with a fluorescence dye. The quantification is performed in real-time [55]. Likewise, there are several other variants of PCR, such as restriction fragment length polymorphism (RFLP) or terminal restriction fragment length polymorphism (t-RFLP) that have been employed to identify the genetic fingerprints available in pathogenic bacteria as well as to achieve microbial profiling for rapid and sensitive detection [56,57].

With several modifications, PCR has already become one of the most trusted conventional molecular diagnostic assays. But the use of thermocycler to adjust the temperature for different steps such as denaturation, annealing, and extension makes it expensive and time-consuming along with other limitations of PCR [58–60].

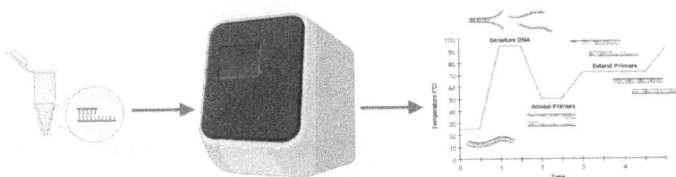

Fig. 1.3 PCR based molecular detection of pathogenic bacteria as one of the most reliable conventional techniques

1.1.5 DNA microarrays technique and whole-genome sequencing (WGS)

DNA microarray profiling is one of the recent advancements in the molecular diagnosis of pathogenic bacteria. It involves immobilizing a designed capture probe to bind with the complementary sequence of template DNA with the detection limit of 10-1000 DNA copies (Fig. 1.4). It can also identify multiple pathogenic bacteria simultaneously and reduces the time for detection remarkably. DNA microarray technology is a large-scale multiplexed technology based on the immobilized probe with different sequences to target a broad range of microorganisms[61,62]. This also helps in differentiating between closely related pathogenic bacteria with the details of genera and species. However, the major drawback with the DNA microarray system is high laboratory expenses in terms of equipment, reagents, and power consumption [63].

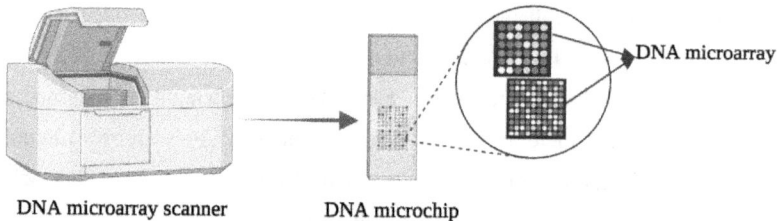

DNA microarray scanner   DNA microchip

Fig. 1.4 DNA microarray profiling

WGS provides information starting from the detection of microbes to identifying the outbreaks. The amount of information provided by WGS in the current diagnosis has made a remarkable stride in improving the sensitivity and curbing false-negative results. However, the drawback associated with WGS is similar to DNA microarray technique due to expensive instruments, reagents, and power consumption [64].

1.1.6 Immunoassay

Immunoassay is based on the interaction between antigens and antibodies with high specificity. In this technique, the concentration of sample analytes can be estimated by measuring the intensity of the resulting colour after the antigen-antibody reaction. The fast diagnosis and facile testing make immunoassay such as Enzyme-Linked Immunosorbent Assay (ELISA) one of the most explored conventional diagnostic techniques to date [65–67]. The pathogenic bacteria have been extensively detected in clinical samples using immunoassay such as sandwich ELISA (Fig. 1.5) with acceptable sensitivity and selectivity [68–72]. However, the cost of immunoassay is a major limitation in providing affordable testing for the diseases caused by pathogenic bacteria [73–75].

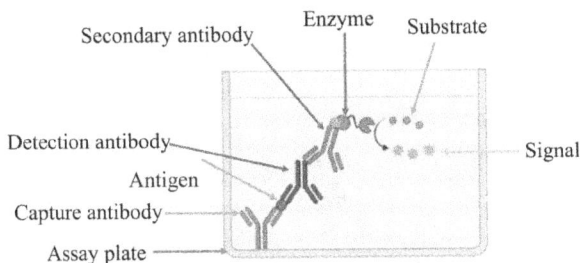

Fig. 1.5 A typical sandwich ELISA for the detection of pathogenic bacteria

1.1.7 Bacteriophage based detection

Bacteriophage is a virus and commonly infects bacterial cells such as *E. coli* and *S.aureus*. The same principle is used for developing the detection assay using bacteriophages to infect the specific bacteria. The identification of pathogenic bacteria is possible with bacteriophage due to its capacity to infect specific bacteria with low cell numbers and improve sensitivity. The traditional method of pathogenic bacteria detection is the plaque method, where the cell culture grown on a Petri plate was analyzed to check the activity of bacteriophage against specific pathogenic bacteria, as shown in Fig. 1.6. This is also called as bacteriophage-typing method [76,77]. However, pathogenic bacteria detection can also be achieved by infecting the bacterial cells with phage by entering into the lysogen life cycle, not allowing cells to burst.

The significant disadvantages of phage-based detection techniques are the time required for assay, unavoidable cross-reactivity, non-specific data, false-positive results, and low detection limit of pathogenic bacteria [78].

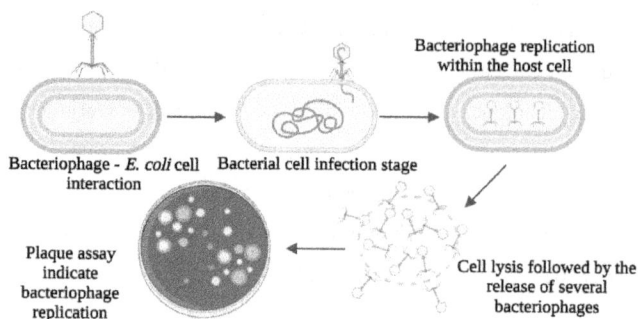

Fig. 1.6 Phage based detection of pathogenic bacteria

Therefore, the drawbacks of existing diagnostic techniques demand an urgent need to develop a promising alternative to address the undeniable problems. The recent advancement shows that a rapid diagnostic test (RDT) might be a fitting substitute for the traditional bacterial diagnostic assays. However, developing RDT that is rapid, precise, robust, sensitive, multiplexed, automated, and cost-effective is a challenge. Several biosensors were developed to address this challenge. In this section, we discuss the basics of biosensors and their type for detecting pathogenic bacteria.

1.2 Biosensors

Biosensors are analytical devices with a biorecognition element specific to the target and a physicochemical transducer that converts the biorecognition event into a measurable signal. A schematic representation of the biosensor is shown in Fig. 1.7. The signal obtained is proportional to the selective binding or interaction of the target with the biorecognition element. The fascinating features of biosensors include rapid analysis, robustness, high sensitivity and selectivity, reliability, low cost, and user-friendly [79–84].

Several strategies have been employed to develop biosensors by varying the transducers and bio-recognition element to investigate real and clinical samples [85–87]. Three categories of the most commonly employed biosensors, viz., i. optical, ii. electrochemical, and iii. mechanical are discussed below.

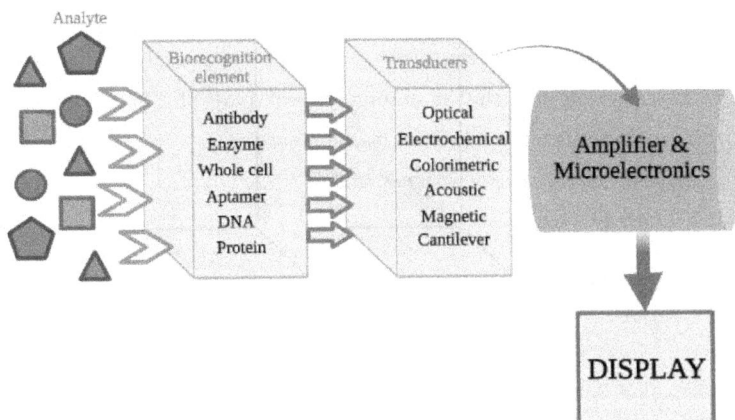

Fig.1.7 Schematic diagram of a typical biosensor

1.2.1 Optical biosensors

The optical sensors monitor the analyte interaction with the bio-recognition element leading to a change in the optical characteristics of the sensors [88,89]. The signals produced from the sensor can be used directly or after amplification. Different detection strategies such as colourimetry, fluorescence, chemiluminescence, surface plasmon resonance (SPR), and surface-enhanced Raman spectroscopy (SERS) have been used for optical biosensing [90–93]. Various optical sensors developed for the detection of pathogenic bacteria are mentioned in Table 1.1.

1.2.1.1 SPR biosensors

SPR is considered an efficient tool to monitor the interaction of target analytes and bio-recognition elements. SPR has been majorly reported in thin metallic films (such as gold layer on the sensor surface) and at the interface between media of different refractive indices. Across the junction of the medium, such as glass and sample solution (lower refractive index), the total internal reflected light escapes as an evanescent wave field. A characteristic absorption spectrum of evanescent wave energy exhibits an SPR dip at a specific incident angle. Similarly, localized SPR (LSPR) sensing is carried out using metallic nanoparticles (e.g., gold nanoparticles) wherein the size of the nanoparticle should be lesser than the wavelength of light

9

[94,95]. The bio-recognition element immobilized over the surface of gold nanoparticles (AuNP) selectively detects the target analyte (like proteins, nucleic acids), resulting in a shift in absorption peak [96]. SPR based optical sensors have been used for detecting different bacteria such as *E. coli* O157:H7, *S. choleraesuis*, *S. typhimurium*, *L. monocytogenes*, and *C. jejuni* with LOD in the range of 10^2 to 10^4 CFU mL^{-1} [97–99].

1.2.1.2 SERS biosensors

Surface-enhanced Raman spectroscopy (SERS) is a powerful tool for biomarker detection because of its ultrahigh detection sensitivity and unique fingerprinting spectra [100,101]. In this technique, the intensity of the vibration spectra of a molecule is enhanced by several orders of magnitude when it is close to nano-roughened metallic surfaces or nanoparticles made of gold or silver [93,102–104]. Table 1.1 highlights some of the optical sensors based on SERS and its modifications for detecting Gram-negative and Gram-positive bacteria like *S. typhimurium*, *B. subtilis* spores and *E. coli* O157:H7 with detection range 10^2-10^7 CFU mL^{-1}.

1.2.1.3 Chemiluminescence biosensors

Chemiluminescence biosensors work on the phenomena of light emission resulting from a chemical reaction. It occurs due to a catalytic reaction, which disintegrates the chemically excited compound to the ground state, resulting in photon emission. The measured light intensity is proportional to the analyte concentration. The leverages provided by such biosensors are many, like high signal-to-noise ratio and easy to use. The non-specific signals can be reduced substantially due to the generation of photons that ensues in the dark by a chemical reaction [105]. A chemiluminescent microarray chip based on polyclonal antibodies was developed for the parallel detection of *E. coli* O157:H7, *S. typhimurium*, and *Legionella pneumophila* [106]. The limitations related to chemiluminescence-based optical biosensors are low signal intensity, poor sensitivity, and cross-reactivity [107].

1.2.1.4 Colourimetric biosensors

Colourimetric detection has contributed immensely to the identification and quantification of pathogenic bacteria. It depends on the interaction between the bio-recognition element and bacteria, resulting in a colour change [108,109]. The advantages associated with colourimetric biosensors include good sensitivity, portability, rapid response, and robustness. Recent advances in colourimetric sensing of bacteria focus on the surface-modified nanoparticles with enhanced sensitivity and selectivity for rapid detection in resource-limited settings [110]. One such approach was reported wherein a colourimetric method was developed using a platinum-coated magnetic nanoparticle cluster to detect *E. coli* with a detection limit as low as 10 CFU mL^{-1} [111].

1.2.1.5 Fluorescence biosensors

The fluorescence-based biosensors depend on the light generated due to electron relaxation from the excited electronic state to the ground state. The bio-recognition elements can be used with and without labels to develop sensitive and selective fluorescence-based optical sensors to detect pathogenic bacteria [112,113].

Fluorescent labeling method involves excitation of the fluorophore at specific wavelength and emission of photons at a different wavelength. These labels are specifically used during the low analyte concentration in the sample under screening [114]. Labeled fluorescence sensors are based on fluorimetric labels such as calcein blue, fluorescent diacetate, and fluorescein isothiocyanate (FITC) [115,116]. These fluorescent dyes can quantify the pathogenic bacteria by labeling the cells directly [117,118]. The blue colour fluorescent dye, calcein, was used for pathogen detection and quantification [119,120]. However, these dyes are harmful, toxic, non-compatible, and photosensitive [116,121]. Therefore, to mitigate the limitations of the conventional fluorescent dyes, nanoparticles such as quantum dots, SWCNT, MWCNT, and carbon dots have been tested [122–124].

Table 1.1: Optical sensors for the detection of pathogenic bacteria

S. No.	Optical sensors	Pathogenic bacteria	Detection range (CFU mL⁻¹)	LOD (CFU mL⁻¹)	Ref.
1	Fluorescein diacetate (FDA) labeled optical sensor	*S. aureus*	—	—	[117]
2	FITC-labeled aptamers based optical biosensor	*P. aeruginosa*	10^2 - 10^3	5.07	[118]
3	Antibody-labeled fiber optic biosensor (FOBS)	*L. monocytogenes, E. coli* and *S. enterica*	10^4 - 10^5	10^3	[125]
4	Label-free antibody functionalized optical sensor	*S. typhimurium*	500 - 5000	247	[126]
5	Wavelength division multiplexing based SPR biosensor	*E. coli* O157:H7 *S. choleraesuis* serotype *typhimurium,* *L. monocytogenes* *C. jejuni*	-	1.4×10^4 4.4×10^4 3.5×10^3 1.1×10^5	[127]
6	ssDNA immobilized SPR biosensor	*S. typhimurium*	10^2 - 10^{10}	10^2	[128]

S. No.	Optical sensors	Pathogenic bacteria	Detection range $(CFU\ mL^{-1})$	LOD $(CFU\ mL^{-1})$	Ref.
7	Silver film over nanosphere substrate-based SERS biosensor	*B. subtilis* spores	—	2.6×10^3	[129]
8	Gold nanoparticle coated starch magnetic bead-based SERS biosensor	*E. coli*	$10^0 - 10^5$	1	[130]
9	Aptamer based SERS biosensor	*E. coli*	$10^2 - 10^6$	10^2	[131]
10	Hemin-Encapsulated Mesoporous Silica Nanoparticles based Chemiluminescence biosensor	*E. coli* and *S. aureus*	$10^1 - 10^9$	3 and 2.5	[132]
11	Multiplexed sandwich immunoassay based Chemiluminescence biosensor	*E. coli*	$8.5 \times 10^4 - 3.7 \times 10^6$	1.8×10^4	[106]
		L. pneumophila	$1.4 \times 10^6 - 2.2 \times 10^7$	7.9×10^4	
		S. typhimurium	$5.0 \times 10^7 - 1.1 \times 10^9$	2.0×10^7	
12	Protein capped nanoparticle based Colourimetric biosensor	*B. subtilis*	$7.5 \times 10^3 - 1.5 \times 10^5$	2.57×10^3	[133]

1.2.2 Electrochemical biosensors

Electrochemical sensors work by detecting the changes in electrical parameters like current, voltage, or impedance of the electrode upon binding with target analytes and are used for qualitative and quantitative estimation [134]. The electrochemical sensors can be classified as amperometric, voltammetric, conductometric, and impedimetric [135–137]. Electrochemical biosensors are the most successful sensors that have achieved both research-oriented and commercial success [138–142]. Of late, screen-printed carbon electrode (SPCE) has emerged as a high throughput sensor that could be deployed as an integral part of Point-of-Care testing (POCT) devices [143–146]. A brief discussion of electrochemical sensors for the detection of pathogenic bacteria is given in the following sections. Table 1.2 presents the different electrochemical biosensors developed for the sensitive and selective detection of pathogenic bacteria.

1.2.2.1 Amperometric biosensors

Amperometric biosensors function at a particular potential difference applied between working and reference electrodes. An oxidation-reduction reaction is activated by the applied potential difference on the surface of the electrode resulting in electric current [147–150]. The generated current intensity is directly proportional to the concentration of the target analyte [151,152]. The most promising factors of amperometric biosensors are simplicity, ease of miniaturization, and excellent sensitivity [147,153,154]. Among various amperometric sensors developed for the detection of pathogenic bacteria, a few have been designed for sensing bacteria such as *E. coli* and *Salmonella spp.* with a detection limit of 10^3 to 10^5 CFU mL^{-1} [155,156].

1.2.2.2 Potentiometric biosensors

Potentiometric biosensor uses ion-selective electrodes to sense the potential difference due to the specific interactions with ions in the sample [157–160]. They have many applications in sensing bioanalytes, including pathogenic bacteria such as *E. coli* and *S. aureus* with a reasonable detection limit of 10^2 and 1 CFU mL^{-1}, respectively [161,162].

1.2.2.3 Impedimetric biosensors

The impedimetric biosensors are based on impedance measurement, which is the resistance to the flow of current in an electric circuit [163–166]. Electrochemical impedance spectroscopy (EIS) is used to study the change in impedance or the charge transfer resistance (R_{ct}) occurring at the electrode-electrolyte interface after the analyte interaction [163,167–169]. In the case of bacterial analysis, impedance microbiology (IM) has been explored to monitor the growth of bacteria by analyzing the change in ionic metabolites [170,171]. With the complexity of bacterial cells and their properties, electrochemical detection may also become tedious to understand. The bacterial cell wall consists of polar heads and hydrophobic non-polar tails. This nature of the bacterial cell wall makes the cell insulating in nature (estimated conductivity is 10^{-7} S m^{-1}). This insulating nature of bacterial cell membranes increases the impedance at the electrode-electrolyte interface [167,172,173]. This is due to the hindrance of the redox-active molecules at the electrode surface after bacterial binding cells [167].

Table 1.2: Electrochemical sensors for pathogen detection

S. No.	Electrochemical sensors	Pathogenic bacteria	Linear Range (CFU mL^{-1})	LOD (CFU mL^{-1})	Ref.
1	Antibody immobilized amperometric biosensor	*Salmonella spp.*	—	~5×10^4	[155]
2	Phage based amperometric biosensor	*Bacillus cereus* and *Mycobacterium smegmatis*	10 - 1000	10	[174]
3	Amperometric magnetoimmuno sensor	*S. aureus*	$1.0 - 1.0\times10^7$	1	[175]
4	SWCNT based potentiometric	*S. aureus*	$1.3\times10^3 - 10^8$	8.0×10^2	[162]

S. No.	Electrochemical sensors	Pathogenic bacteria	Linear Range (CFU mL^{-1})	LOD (CFU mL^{-1})	Ref.
5	Label free potentiometric immunosensor	*Salmonella spp.*	$13 - 1.3 \times 10^6$	6	[176]
6	Impedimetric immunosensor	*E. coli*	$4 \times 10^3 - 10^6$	4×10^3	[177]
7	Impedimetric immunosensor	*C. jejuni*	1.0×10^3 to 1.0×10^7	1.0×10^3	[178]
8	Impedimetric immunosensor	*E. coli, Streptococcus pyogenes*	$10 - 10^8$ (*E. coli*), $10^4 - 10^7$ (*Streptococcus pyogenes*)	10 and 10^3 (whole and lysed cells)	[179,180]
9	Impedance biosensor chips based on epoxysilanes monolayer	*E. coli*	$6 \times 10^4 - 10^7$	6×10^3	[181]
10	Nanoporous membrane based impedimetric immunosensor	*E. coli*	$10 - 10^5$	10	[182]
11	Aptamer-based impedimetric sensor	*Salmonella typhimurium*	$1 \times 10^3 - 10^5$	600	[183]

1.2.3 Mechanical biosensors

The mechanical biosensor functions on the principle of mass variations by monitoring the minute changes in the mass during the analyte detection [184]. The minute mass variations are monitored using piezoelectric crystals that are made to vibrate at a specific frequency by applying an electric field. Additional mass variations due to the binding of pathogenic bacteria with the bio-recognition element create a change in vibrational frequency. Finally, the change in vibrational/oscillation frequency can be measured electrically, and the variations due to the additional mass of the crystal can be calculated [185,186]. The label-free, relatively low-cost, sensitive, and specific mechanical biosensors are categorized into two major types, i. piezoelectric (such as quartz crystal microbalance (QCM) biosensors and piezoelectric cantilever biosensors) and ii. magnetoelastic (ME) biosensors[163].

1.2.3.1 Piezoelectric methods

1.2.3.1.1 Quartz crystal microbalance (QCM) biosensors

QCM biosensors for pathogen detection have been developed by immobilizing antibodies on the surface of QCM to capture the target pathogen and generate a frequency signal [187–190]. In this context, an immunosensor based on piezoelectric QCM has been reported for the detection of *Salmonella typhimurium*. This was achieved by measuring the resonant frequency and motional resistance simultaneously [191]. The limitations of QCM based biosensors include expensive sensor development procedures, high cross-reactivity, and poor specificity [192].

1.2.3.1.2 Piezoelectric cantilever biosensors

The piezoelectric cantilever biosensors for pathogen detection are based on the response of a sensitive cantilever (or microcantilever) immobilized with bio-recognition elements [193–196]. These cantilevers have a characteristic resonant frequency, and any variations in the cantilever oscillations bring a notable change in the resonant frequency [197,198]. This variation occurs due to the binding of the target analyte with the bio-recognition element [199].

1.2.3.2 Magnetoelastic (ME) sensor

ME sensors are ribbon-like thick film strips derived from amorphous ferromagnetic alloys such as $Fe_{40}Ni_{38}Mo_4B_{18}$ (Metglas 2826MB) [200,201]. These sensors produce longitudinal vibrations when exposed to a gradient magnetic field and, in turn, generate elastic waves. Due to the generation of elastic waves within the magnetoelastic materials, a magnetic flux develops, which can be detected remotely. The sensing mechanism of ME sensor is based on resonance variation due to the change in the surrounding medium. The optical, acoustic, or magnetic techniques have been used for monitoring resonance characteristics of the ME sensor. These ME sensors have been used to measure solution pH and detect several chemical-biological agents such as glucose, ricin, endotoxin B, and pathogenic bacteria like *E. coli* [202].

1.2.4 Bio-recognition elements

The commonly used bio-recognition elements for the development of biosensors are antibodies, enzymes, protein, nucleic acids, enzymes, aptamers, and antibiotics [203–206]. The bio-recognition elements used for specific detection of Gram-positive and negative bacteria are discussed in the following sections.

1.2.4.1 Antibodies

The performance of any biosensor depends on the type of bio-recognition element used for the bio-sensing application. In the case of immunosensors, the performance largely depends upon the type of antibodies and its immobilization approach. Antibodies are brilliant bio-recognition elements due to the higher sensitivity and specificity against the cognate antigen and are considered the ideal candidate for integration into sensors [207,208]. The performance of the antibody-based biosensor depends on the three factors; i. ability to immobilize antibodies without losing their natural activity, ii. accessibility of the antibodies towards the target analyte, and iii. minimum non-specific adsorption to the solid support [209]. Based on these criteria, antibodies have been immobilized covalently and non-covalently for the sensing of bio-analytes such as pathogenic bacteria. Several antibodies based optical and impedimetric immunosensors have been developed for the detection of pathogenic bacteria [210–214].

1.2.4.2 Nucleic acids

Nucleic acids such as DNA/RNA-based biosensors are also known as genosensors. It works on the principle of complementary binding of probe DNA to the specific target DNA. The complementary probe DNA can be designed on the basis of nucleotide sequences present on target DNA [215,216]. These complementary probes are immobilized at the sensor surface as a bio-recognition element. The specific detection of the target DNA strand can be achieved based on the unique recognition pattern available on the complementary probe. Of late, various nucleic acid-based bio-recognition element has been reported such as locked nucleic acid (LNA) and peptide nucleic acid (PNA) for the detection of pathogenic bacteria [207].

1.2.4.3 Enzymes

The enzyme catalyzes the specific substrate into a product resulting in a measurable output that includes protons, electrons, light, and heat. The enzymes have been incorporated with the optical, electrochemical, and colorimetric transducers to detect target analytes such as pathogenic bacteria in clinical samples [203,217].

1.2.4.4 Antibiotics

Antibiotics like vancomycin and daptomycin exhibited a specific towards Gram-positive bacteria. These are glycopeptide drugs and can specifically bind with D-Ala-D-Ala part of the small peptide present in the peptidoglycan of the bacterial cell wall [218–220]. Similarly, antibiotics such as polymyxin/colistin are peptide antibiotics group having five derivatives *viz.*, A, B, C, D, and E. The activity of polymyxin is specific to the LPS layer available in the outer membrane of the Gram-negative cell wall. The subunits of the LPS layer are integrated using divalent cations such as Mg^{2+} and Ca^{2+}. The polycationic nature of polymixin replaces the divalent cations when it reaches the close vicinity of the bacterial cell wall. This results in disintegrating the LPS layer leading to pore generation on the cell wall and finally cell lysing. Therefore, polymixin has been used as an effective bio-recognition element for the specific detection of Gram-negative bacteria. For example, polymyxin B was coupled with a cyanine dye by Chen et al. for the specific detection of Gram-negative bacteria [206,221,222].

1.2.4.5 Lectin

Lectins are known carbohydrate-binding proteins that have specific interaction with the sugar moieties. The lectins exhibit a significant affinity for carbohydrates residues like mannose and other polysaccharides present on the surface of Gram-positive and Gram-negative bacteria. Lectins such as Wheat Germ Agglutinin (WGA) and concanavalin A (ConA) were explored to differentiate Gram-positive bacteria from Gram-negative [223,224].

1.2.4.6 Metabolizable compounds

These compounds have been synthesized from various metabolic pathways and are used to label the peptidoglycan layer specifically [225]. The fluorophore-modified bio-orthogonal groups (alkynes, azide, etc.) have been used to attain direct and indirect labeling through a click chemistry reaction [226,227]. The most common procedure for labeling Gram-positive bacteria is the maltodextrin transport mechanism of bacteria. The known metabolic precursor for bacterial labeling is D-amino acids that can be integrated within the peptidoglycan layer of Gram-positive bacterial cell wall. The metabolic precursors coupled with organic and near-infra red fluorophore have been used for labeling [228,229]. In this context, Wang and coworkers used fluorescent D-amino acids labels for labeling and imaging Gram-positive bacteria specifically [230]. For the detection of Gram-negative bacteria, a metabolizable compound viz., 3-deoxy-D-mannose caprylic acid (Kdo), which plays a significant role in the synthesis of the LPS layer, was targeted. Wang et al. labeled Kdo with a developed fluorophore and could detect Gram-negative bacteria specifically [231].

1.2.4.7 Lysozyme

Lysozyme can hydrolyze the β-(1, 4) glycosidic bond between NAG and NAM of the peptidoglycan layer to lyse the cell wall and kill the Gram-positive bacteria. Lysozyme act directly on the cell wall of Gram-positive bacteria (due to thick peptidoglycan) over Gram-negative bacteria [232].

1.2.4.8 Cationic complex

The positively charged cationic platinum (II) potentially binds the negatively charged LPS to develop LPS–Pt(II) aggregates that helps in the specific detection of Gram-negative bacteria [233].

1.2.4.9 Boronic acid

Boronic acid exhibited a selective affinity for cis-diol groups through the formation of cyclic esters. This interaction was used in synthesizing a boronic acid copolymer-poly (4-vinylphenylboronic acid-methyl-2-acrylic acid- (2-dimethylamino) ethyl methyl ester-n-butyl methacrylate) (pVDB)) for the early detection of bacteria such as *E. coli* and *S. aureus* [234]. The interaction is based on reversible boronate-ester formation with glycol-rich sugar residues available on the bacterial membrane.

1.2.4.10 Carbohydrates

The primary carbohydrate sources used for the detection of bacteria are the large sugar residues such as maltose, maltotriose, and malto-hexose. The designed fluorescent probe can use these carbohydrate residues as the bio-recognition element to differentiate bacterial infections from other diseases. In one of the similar approaches, maltotriose was used as a recognition element to synthesize a fluorescence probe for the detection of Gram-negative bacteria [235]. The carbohydrate residue like mannose has a higher affinity to the hair-like projections known as pili. Mannose-based polymers exhibited a strong interaction with the mannose receptors available on the cell wall of Gram-negative bacteria and were used for its detection [236].

1.2.4.11 Aptamers

Aptamers are composed of a single-stranded oligomeric stretch of nucleic acids. They are designed in such a way so that they can bind to the specific proteins or carbohydrate residues available on the surface of the bacterial cell wall. Aptamers, designed using systematic evolution of ligands through exponential enrichment (SELEX), target several entities on the bacterial cell wall. The aptamers in conjugation with nanomaterials have also been used for the specific detection of bacteria [237–240].

1.2.4.12 Biorecognition elements for non-specific detection of bacteria

The biorecognition elements have shown non-covalent interactions with negatively charged bacteria commonly due to electrostatic and hydrophobic effects.

These types of interactions are non-specific in nature. There are several chemical, and biological entities explored for pathogen detection based on non-specific interactions. The small molecule fluorescence probes exhibit aggregation-induced emission (AIE). It is a unique and intriguing photo-physical phenomenon that occurs when the fluorescence molecule aggregates, resulting in the enhancement of fluorescence. Of late, several positively charged AIEgens have been used to identify different bacteria [241, 242]. Antimicrobial peptides (AMP) are known to have amphiphilic positively charged peptide arrangements of several amino acid residues. AMP exhibit both electrostatic and hydrophobic interaction with bacterial cell wall due to the presence of charged polar and non-polar amino acid residues. The electrostatic interaction helps bring AMP in close vicinity to bacterial cell wall and the hydrophobic end of AMP selectively binds with bacteria and penetrates through the cell wall [243].

The significant improvements in bio-recognition element certainly plays a crucial role in the development of bacterial biosensors. Almost all bio-recognition elements possess some unavoidable limitations in terms such as sophisticated handling, cross-reactivity, shelf life, cost and complex pre-enrichment steps [244]. Hence, to attain rapid, cost-effective and accurate detection of pathogenic bacteria need of advanced bio-recognition element such as nanomaterials is inevitable.

1.3 Nanomaterials for the detection of pathogenic bacteria

Nanomaterials are materials possessing at least one dimension in the size range of less than 100 nm. These materials are synthesized in controlled environments so that their properties can be tuned for potential applications [245–247]. The different types of nanomaterials have been discussed below, and various sensors based on nanomaterials have been provided in Table 1.3.

1.3.1 Metal nanoparticles

Metal nanoparticles (MNP) are nanoscale particles made up of pure metals such as gold and silver. It consists of a metal core covered by organic or inorganic/metal or metal oxide shell. The unique characteristics of MNP like SPR, LSPR, and other optical properties make it a promising tool for biosensing applications [248–251]. The extensive usage of MNPs such as gold (Au) and silver

(Ag) nanoparticles for the development of biochemical sensors or pathogen biosensors as chemical "nose" has been explored [252,253]. MNPs exhibit localized SPR, and it depends on the particle size, geometry, and molecular interaction with the surrounding dielectric medium. More than one SPR band is exhibited by different types of AuNP, such as Au nanorods (AuNR), nanobranches, and nano-bipyramids. For example, the Au nanorod projects two SPR bands; one longitudinal band from the visible region to NIR and another transverse band in the visible region only [254].

The colourimetric detection of pathogenic bacteria was achieved using MNPs to improve the specificity and sensitivity by varying their surface area and size. The significant characteristics of MNPs, such as controllable synthesis, excellent solubility, facile surface modification, and excellent biocompatibility, have been explored. The interactions between MNPs and target analyte result in a colour change that can be identified by UV-Vis absorbance spectroscopy [255].

1.3.2 Magnetic nanoparticles

Magnetic nanoparticles (Mag-NP) have unique magnetic properties that find applications in various fields like drug delivery, gene transfer, and pathogen detection [256]. Mag-NPs, like magnetite (Fe_3O_4) or maghemite ($g-Fe_2O_3$) have excellent thermal, chemical, and colloidal stability, making them a promising candidate for bio-sensing. Recently, mono-dispersed Mag-NP has been used to screen the presence of pathogenic bacteria [257].

1.3.3 Conjugated polymer nanoparticles

Conjugated polymers, also known as conducting polymers, have extended π – conjugated backbones and delocalized electronic frameworks. These are widely used in optoelectronic devices like photovoltaic cells, field-effect transistors, light-emitting diodes, and their significant electronic properties make them efficient fluorescence probes. The potential of conjugated polymers, especially water-soluble conjugated polymers (WSCPs), for developing chemical/biological sensors, fluorescence imaging, gene transfer, and drug delivery have been studied [258].

1.3.4 Hybrid/ bimetallic nanoparticles

The properties of these nanoparticles are determined by the metal used for the synthesis and their size. The synergistic effect of two metals has been utilized for specialized applications such as diagnostics and therapeutics [259]. In this context, silicon quantum dots (Si-QDs) and iron-based superparamagnetic iron oxide nanoparticles were combined to explore the diagnostics and therapeutics utilities of hybrid nanoparticles [260]. Likewise, different combinations of nanoparticles have been tested to modulate the intrinsic properties of hybrid nanoparticles to achieve imaging, sensing, and drug delivery [261–263].

Table 1.3: Different nanomaterials used for the detection of pathogenic bacteria

Nanom aterials	Detection type	Target	Sample type	Receptor	LOD	Ref.
AuNR	SPR	E. coli	RO water and coconut water	Lectin-Mannose	10^3 CFU mL^{-1}	[264]
		C. jejuni and C. coli	Stool	ssDNA of cadF gene	10^2 CFU mL^{-1}	[265]
	Colourimetric	S. aureus	Chinese cabbage and beef	Urease and yolk immuno-globulin (IgY)	476 CFU mL^{-1}	[266]
AuNP	Colourimetric	Salmonella spp.	Chicken meat with skin	ssDNA	<10 CFU mL^{-1}	[267]
		E. coli	Standard buffer	Aptamers	1 µg mL^{-1}	[268]

Nanom aterials	Detection type	Target	Sample type	Receptor	LOD	Ref.
AuNP	Colourimetric	*V. parahemolyticus*	Oyster	Polyclonal IgG antibodies	10 CFU mL^{-1}	[269]
Magnetic beads	Chemilumin escent	*S. aureus*	Lake water, milk, human urine and human saliva	Rabbit immuno-globulin G (ALP-IgG)	3.3 CFU mL^{-1}	[270]
	SERS	*E. coli, S. aureus* and *P. aeruginosa*	Blood	AMP	10 CFU mL^{-1}	[271]
Magnetic probes	Colourimetric	*E. coli*	Drinking water	T7 bacterio -phage	10^4 CFU mL^{-1}	[272]
	Fluorimetric	*S. aureus*	Blood	TiO$_2$-coated Mag-NP	10^2 CFU mL^{-1}	[273]
P3HT-b-P3TEGT (Core-shell NPs)	Electrochem ical	*E. coli*	Tap and the Nile water	Poly(3-hexylthiop hene)-b-poly(3-triethylene-glycol-thiophene)	500 CFU mL^{-1}	[274]
Pt–Au NPs	Colourimetric	*E. coli*	Standard buffer	TMB–H$_2$O$_2$ peroxidase	10^2 CFU mL^{-1}	[275]
Au@Pt NP/SiO$_2$	Immunoassay	*E. coli*	Milk samples	Monoclona l Antibodies	2.16 × 10^2 CFU mL^{-1}	[276]

1.3.5 Fluorescent nanoparticles

In biological samples, fluorescent nanoparticles are generally utilized for marking processes in living cells. These nanoparticles emit fluorescence after absorbing light of a specific wavelength. It has recently emerged as a promising tool for several applications, especially in targeted drug delivery, gene transfer, sensing bio-analytes, and bacterial cell imaging [277–281]. The fluorescent nanoparticles (FNP) such as quantum dots (QDs) and carbon-based nanomaterials (carbon dots) have exhibited interesting properties such as tunable photoluminescent (PL) emission, resistance to photobleaching, biocompatibility, and nontoxicity[282,283].

1.3.5.1 Quantum dots

A relatively new class of nanoparticles, quantum dots (QDs), have been used as an efficient colourimetric and fluorescent probe to detect pathogenic bacteria. They are nanoscale semiconductor crystals with a size of less than 10 nm. The composition of QDs are as follows: a) a core with group II-VI atoms such as cadmium selenide (CdSe) or group III-V atoms like indium phosphide, b) a shell surrounding the core which is mainly made up of zinc sulphide (ZnS), to enhance the optical properties, improve stability and decrease cytotoxicity and c) a capping layer to convert QDs into the hydrophilic compound to attach with biomolecules like peptide, proteins, nucleic acids, oligonucleotide and tiny molecules [284]. The size variation in QDs exhibits emission of a different colour due to a change in the bandgap. QDs are a better alternative to organic fluorescent dyes because of their broad absorption range, tunable photoluminescence, longer fluorescent lifetime, higher surface-to-volume ratio, and resistance to photobleaching [285]. Hence, QDs had been actively used as a suitable nanoprobe to detect bacteria such as *E. coli* O157:H7, *S. typhimurium*, *L. monocytogenes*, *V. parahaemolyticus* [286–289]. The disadvantages of using QDs, especially with the biological samples, are the biocompatibility issues and cytotoxic nature. Hence, there is an urgent need to replace conventional QDs with biocompatible and non-toxic quantum dots.

Recently, carbon dots have emerged as a class of biocompatible and non-toxic fluorescent probes with remarkable properties for live-cell imaging. The thesis work focuses entirely on carbon dots and their application to detect pathogenic bacteria. Therefore, we have discussed carbon dots, synthesis strategies, and type of carbon dots, photoluminescence mechanism, spectroscopic properties, and surface functionalization/ passivation as a separate section.

1.4 Carbon dots

In pursuit of a non-toxic, biocompatible, photostable, and highly tunable multicolour fluorescent nanoprobe, serendipitously discovered carbon dots (CDs) emerged as a potential solution. CDs are a budding class of fluorescent nanomaterials having quasi-spherical morphology with a size range from 0 to 10 nm. It was first synthesized in 2004 as a purified by-product of single-walled carbon nanotubes (SWCNT) [290]. The physicochemical properties of CDs resemble their contemporary semiconductor quantum dots (QD) [291]. CDs could replace the traditional QD in bacterial cell imaging mainly due to four reasons; (i) the solubility and stability of CDs, (ii) biocompatibility of CDs towards living cells, (iii) photostability of CDs even with longtime irradiation of light, different temperatures, pH and ionic conditions, and (iv) cost-effective and scalable synthesis procedures [292–297], [303-328].

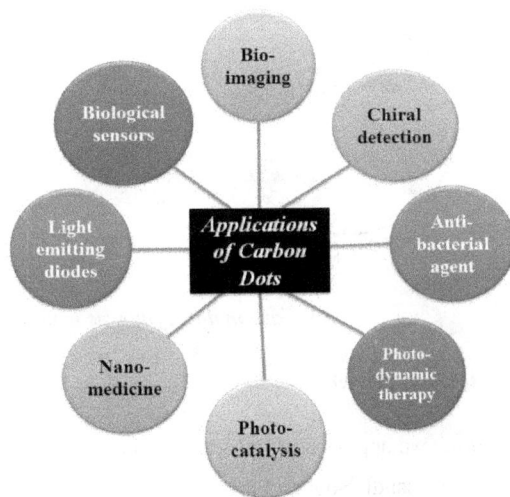

Fig 1.8 Different applications of carbon dots

27

Carbon dots are widely employed in various fields, like drug delivery, nanomedicine, photo-dynamic therapy, photo-catalysis, antibacterial agent, bio-sensing, and bio-imaging, schematically shown in Fig. 1.8. Therefore, a thorough understanding of the different properties of CDs, including their emission mechanism, along with their synthesis techniques, is required to design and develop optical and electrochemical biosensors.

1.4.1 Carbon dots synthesis strategies

The synthesis methods of CDs have evolved from the conventional arc-discharge method to the recent microwave-assisted synthesis. The synthesis strategies of CDs have been split into two major categories *viz*; top-down and bottom-up approaches [292,298–301], as shown in Fig. 1.9.

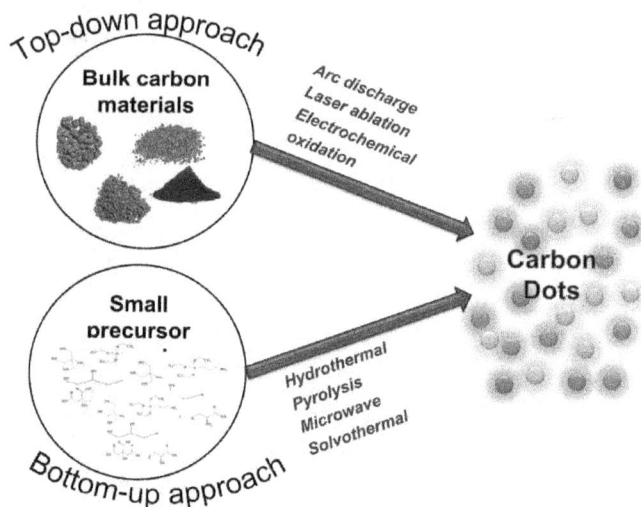

Fig. 1.9 Carbon dots synthesis methods

1.4.1.1 Top-down approach

The top-down approach of CD synthesis depends on breaking complex carbon precursors such as candle soot and graphite powder into smaller and simpler carbon nanodots. The top-down method of CD synthesis includes arc discharge, laser ablation, acid oxidation, and electrochemical synthesis [292,299,300,302–304].

28

In the arc discharge method, a bulk carbon material is taken as the anode. The carbon material is decomposed by gas plasma at high temperatures (up to 4000 K). The carbon vapour generated due to high temperature assembles at the cathode to form CD. The CD synthesized by this method has a relatively large size which reduces the surface area, thus limiting the active fluorescent centers [305].

CDs were synthesized using the laser ablation technique by Sun et al., wherein the high-energy laser was irradiated onto a carbon target. Due to high temperature and pressure, the target heats up instantly and evaporates into a plasma state. The vapours then crystallize to form CD while cooling. The CD synthesized from this method exhibit narrow size distribution, good water solubility, photostability, and non-blinking fluorescence [306].

In the acid oxidation method, the bulk carbon material is treated with acid to exfoliate and decompose into carbon nanoparticles. Due to acid oxidation, several functional groups such as hydroxyl or carboxyl groups are available on the surface of CD resulting in improved hydrophilicity. The synthesized CDs have a narrow size distribution, high photoluminescence, and good photostability [307].

The electrochemical method of CD synthesis is based on the exfoliation of carbon electrodes by applying a potential. Bulk carbon materials like graphite rod, graphite powder, carbon fibers, and multi-walled carbon nanotubes (MWCNT) are commonly used as the carbon electrode source in electrolytes like sodium hydroxide, phosphate buffer solution, and potassium persulfate [308,309].

1.4.1.2 Bottom-up approach

The bottom-up approach for CD synthesis has been extensively used due to low-cost, large-scale synthesis and facile methodology. This synthesis approach includes combustion/thermal oxidation, hydrothermal/solvothermal, and microwave-assisted methods [310,311]. Hydrothermal synthesis of carbon dots is carried out in a furnace using precursors such as small organic compounds or polymers with water as the solvent. The obtained CDs have prominent optical and electronic properties, such as high photostability with non-blinking PL emission. The hydrothermally synthesized CD particles are monodispersed and uniformly spherical with a high quantum yield [312–314]. Zhu et al. demonstrated the synthesis of an efficient CD-based nanoprobe with a uniform size distribution emitting bright fluorescence and excellent quantum yield (80%) [315]. Likewise, various CDs with acceptable quantum yield, biocompatibility, tunability, and non-toxic properties were synthesized using a one-pot facile hydrothermal method with different precursor combinations [316–320]. In the solvothermal synthesis of CD, solvents like Dimethyl formamide (DMF), glycol, formamide, and ethanol are commonly used instead of water [321–324].

The other reported bottom-up approaches for synthesizing CD include template-assisted methods, reverse micelle and green chemistry techniques. The template-assisted synthesis involves hard and soft templates with different organic precursors as a carbon source [325]. The reverse micelles are nano-sized water droplets formed due to the action of surfactants dissolved in water with inverse polarity. These reverse micelles can act as a nanoreactor for the synthesis of CD [326]. Green chemistry uses natural precursors like cabbage, papaya, peanut shell, potato starch, *Ocimum sanctum*, egg white, lemon, watermelon, pomegranate, citrus, gram, and garlic for CD synthesis, eliminating the need for chemical precursors. These CDs find applications in heavy metal detection, bio-imaging, detection, drug and gene delivery [327–341].

1.4.2 Types of CDs

CD has been classified into four main categories based on carbon core, size and structure. Fig. 1.10 shows the different types of CDs such as graphene quantum dots, carbon quantum dots, carbon nanodots, and carbon polymer dots [342].

1.4.2.1 Graphene quantum dots

Graphene quantum dots (GQDs) is a zero-dimensional nanomaterial having photoluminescence property. They are small graphene fragments with single or multiple graphene sheets where the size varies from 3 to 20 nm [343,344]. They show excellent physicochemical properties due to interlayer defects and possess quantum confinement, surface passivation, and edge effect. GQDs with a higher degree of oxidation results in extended conjugated π domains that act as the photoluminescence centers. The brilliant electronic properties of GQDs, biocompatible nature, and low cost of preparation make it superior to semiconductor quantum dots [345]. GQDs also has good thermal and electrical conductivity because of the availability of π–π electrons in the sp² hybridized graphene. The low quantum yield reported in GQDs limits their applications for optical-based bacterial sensing [346].

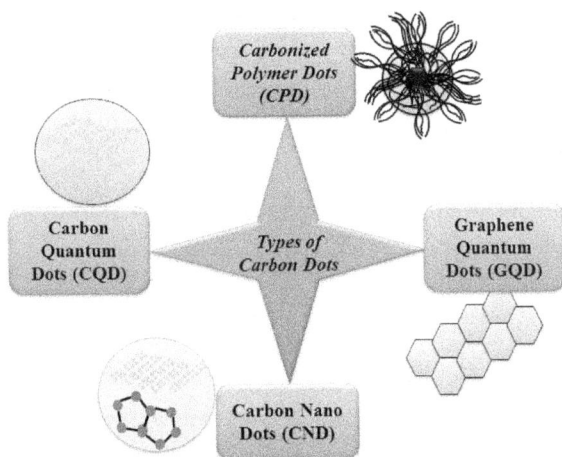

Fig. 1.10 Types of carbon dots

1.4.2.2 Carbon quantum dots

Carbon quantum dots (CQDs) are zero-dimensional nanomaterial with a uniform spherical shape [347, 348]. The size-dependent fluorescence tuning in CQDs is due to quantum confinement as the average particles size ranges from 1 to 4 nm. It also consists of crystal lattices with definite interatomic distances. CQD solution appears transparent in daylight and has a bright fluorescence at a certain excitation wavelength [349,350].

1.4.2.3 Carbon nanodots

The carbon nanodots (CNDs) were synthesized as a by-product of purified SWCNT exhibiting a strong blue fluorescence. CNDs are carbon-based amorphous nanoparticles with a size < 10 nm [351]. During the synthesis of CNDs, carbon precursors undergo nucleation, carbonization (for the synthesis of carbon core), and thermal oxidation for surface passivation. The photoluminescent centers originate from the defect/surface state within the carbon core of CNDs [352].

1.4.2.4 Carbon polymer dots (CPDs)

CPDs are a relatively new type of carbon dots consisting of a carbon core and surface with abundant functional group/ polymer chain. According to Xia et al., the carbon core of CPDs can be classified into four; (i) completely carbonized core as in CQD, (ii) completely carbonized core as in CND, (iii) a carbon core surrounded by polymer frames with a paracrystalline carbon structure and (iv) a cross-linked carbon core with the close-knit polymer frame structure. CPDs photoluminescence centers originate due to surface functionalities and polymer cross-link enhanced emission (CEE) [353,354].

1.4.3 Spectroscopic properties of carbon dots

1.4.3.1 UV-Vis spectroscopy

UV-Vis absorption is an important spectroscopic analysis to find the excitation wavelength used for the electronic transition from the ground state to an excited state. The UV-Vis absorption peaks for CD generally occur at a lower wavelength (250-300 nm), which corresponds to the π-π^* transition of sp^2 conjugated carbon domain. The second peak, usually seen at a higher wavelength (>300 nm), is attributed to the n-π^* transition [355,356]. CDs under UV lamps typically exhibit bright blue colour emission, but green and red colour emissions have also been reported [357,358].

1.4.3.2 Photoluminescence

The PL of CD has been investigated meticulously due to its brilliant spectral properties. The excitation-dependent emission is one of the major intrinsic properties of CDs. The bathochromic or hypsochromic shift can be clearly observed as excitation wavelength changes. The PL emission mechanism is hypothesized using several concepts such as quantum confinement, surface passivation resulting in emissive trap sites and edge effects, heteroatomic doping, and radiative recombination [295,359].

1.4.4 Theoretical implications for PL emission of CD

The origin of PL and its characteristics in CD is poorly understood and still remains uncertain. The different theories to explain the important PL emission features of CD such as high quantum yield, low photobleaching, no fluorescence blinking and excitation dependent emission have been reported [323] and discussed in the following sections.

1.4.4.1 Quantum confinement

Quantum confinement is one of the most accepted theories for validation of PL emission in CDs. The quantum confinement of CDs exhibits a similar trend of size-based light emission as in traditional quantum dots [360]. The organic CD having graphene carbon core with surface functionalities believed to possess intrinsic PL center because of conjugated π-domains. The Density Functional Theory (DFT) calculations for the energy gap between HOMO and LUMO for a benzene ring was ~7 eV, which reduces to ~2 eV for CDs with 20 aromatic rings as shown in Fig. 1.11A. Hence, the PL emission of CD can be tuned by adjusting the energy gap with size variations of conjugated π-domains. The unique blue shift emission was observed when the size of CD particle gets smaller[342,361,362].

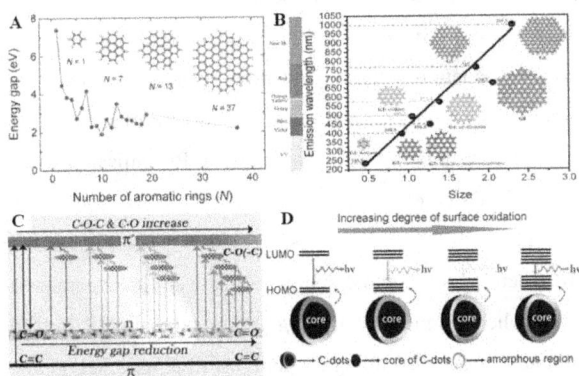

Fig. 1.11 Mechanistic implications of PL emission of carbon dots based on A) energy gap corresponding to π–π^* transitions as a function of the number of aromatic rings B) variations in the size of the carbon dots C) different oxygen-containing surface functional groups (tunable emission) D) increase in the degree of surface oxidation (proposed model based on DFT calculations) [363,364]

The quantum confinement effect is observed when the size of the CD is smaller than the Bohr's exciton radius. The nonzero energy gap of CD can tune the PL emission by varying the size of the particles as shown in Fig. 1.11B. Moreover, different surface edge configurations such as localized zig-zag, and arm-chair edge exhibit variation in quantum confinement due to changes in the energy gap [363,364].

1.4.4.2 Surface passivation

Sun et al. in 2006 had reported that the PL emission in CDs was due to surface passivation. Since then, many organic, inorganic, polymers, and biological entities have been used by researchers to control PL emission by surface passivation. The emissive nature of CDs can be attributed to two main reasons: (a) intrinsic emission due to the size of the sp^2 carbon core and (b) surface passivation achieved by functional groups such as hydroxyl, amide, carboxyl, and carbonyl moieties as shown in Fig. 1.11C. Surface passivation or surface functionalization is the process of introducing defects by incorporating functional groups on the surface of CDs. Sun et al. and Ray et al. had used nitric acid treatment to initialize surface oxidation on CDs. This was considered to be an efficient chemical route for incorporating nitrogen and oxygen atoms into the carbon moieties of CD [365]. Moreover, surface oxidation creates several emissive trap sites by incorporating different functional groups. These emissive traps contain numerous excitons made up of electrons and holes. When the photo-induced electrons present in the emissive trap site move out to recombine with a complementary hole, a bright and glowing PL emission was observed. The optical properties of CDs can be manipulated by reducing oxygen functional groups and can be displayed by different PL emission patterns. The PL emission of CDs recorded a red shift when hydroxyl and epoxide groups were incorporated on the surface of CDs. Therefore, when the number of oxygen groups available on the CD surface is higher, the bandgap is reduced, leading to the red shift (Fig. 1.11D) [366–369].

The tuning of PL emission in CDs can also be attributed to the surface edge defects, such as zig-zag or arm-chair, induced by the passivating agents. The DFT and Time-Dependent DFT (TDDFT) calculations suggest a smaller energy gap (0.14 eV) for zig-zag than for arm-chair edges (0.34 eV). It was observed that the localized

34

states in zig-zag edged CDs moved towards the edge sites, while in arm-chair edged CDs, the localized states are dispersed in the center. Therefore, the smaller energy gap zig-zag edged CDs exhibited a red shift, and the arm-chair edged CDs with larger energy/bandgap displayed a blue shift. The carbene-like structure of zig-zag edges usually consists of a triplet ground state, while the arm-chair exhibits a carbine-like structure with a singlet state [363].

1.4.4.3 Heteroatomic doping

The PL emission mechanism was also explained based on heteroatomic doping, in which PL emission is enhanced by modulating the electronic properties of CD. The doping in the carbon framework can be achieved by in-plane substitution, intercalation, and surface replacement. A dopant with higher electronegativity creates energy states with a higher bandgap and hence exhibits blue PL emission. On the other hand, a dopant with lower electronegativity creates an energy level with a lower bandgap and shows PL emission spectra with a red shift. The content of dopants can be tuned by varying the proportion of the precursors used for CD synthesis, which regulates intrinsic properties such as QY and PL emission [370].

The heteroatomic doping of CDs can be classified as n-type and p-type based on the majority of charge carriers (electrons and holes). The nitrogen (N) atom is one of the most used n-type dopants to tune the PL emission response in CDs. The nitrogen-doped CD (N-CD) shows blue PL emission because N atom is an electron acceptor, due to which the bandgap increases within the HOMO-LUMO orbital. Similarly, the phosphorus (P) atom is another n-type dopant that influences the electronic properties of CDs. P atom is responsible for increasing the defect inside the carbon framework of P doped CDs resulting in bandgap variations and hence tuning of PL emission [371].

Unlike nitrogen, the sulphur (S) atom is an electron donor with no remarkable difference in the electronegativity of S (2.58) and C (2.55) atoms. This results in compromised charge transfer between C-S composite, due to which the introduction of S atom into the CD framework becomes difficult. The p-type doping also modulates the spectral properties of CDs. The p-type dopants such as boron act as electron acceptors, which results in generating holes/positive charges. The formation of holes creates additional electronic transitions, leading to bandgap variations; therefore, the PL emission can be tuned [372].

The co-doping strategies were used extensively to enhance the PL emission response. This is due to the synergistic effect of radiative recombination of trapped electron-hole pairs from multiple emissive sites and energy trap states. The several co-doping strategies have been employed to obtained CD with high quatum yield, bright and tunable PL emission and higher photostability. The co-doping approaches such as N-S co-doped CD with excellent quantum yield was obtained by Dong et al. and was compared with single doped carbon dots such as O-doped and N-doped carbon dots. It was observed that N-S co-doped CD was emitting fluorescence with highest quantum yield (73%) [373]. Similarly, Ding and co-workers used α-lipoic acid with sodium hydroxide and ethylenediamine to obtained N-S co-doped CD with strong blue PL emission with 54.4% quantum yield and used for sensing Fe^{+3} ions [374]. Likewise, N-P and N-B co-doping strategies have exploited for various applications such as heavy metal sensing, bio-imaging, and many more [375,376].

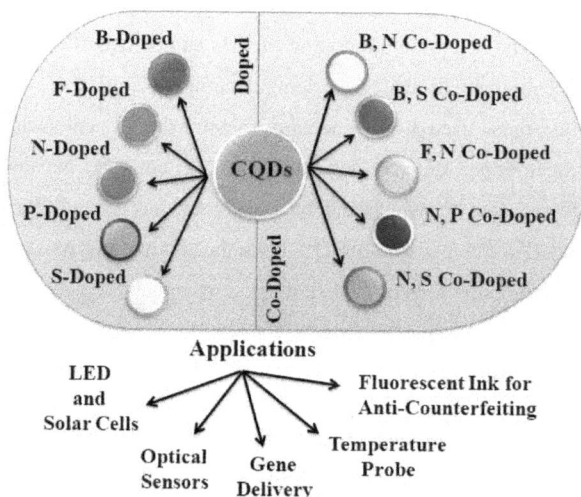

Fig. 1.12 Doping strategies of carbon dots using single or multiple atoms and their applications[377]

1.4.4.4 Radiative recombination

Since the inception of CDs, the concept of radiative recombination has been used effectively to explain the PL emission response [306]. The radiative transition of the conduction band electron to the valence band hole is emitted in the form of a photon. This process is initiated only when the electron absorbs a photon having energy higher than the bandgap of the semiconductor in the valence band. This results in an electron shift to the conduction band. The emitted photon dissipates energy in the form of light, and hence the photoluminescence is observed.

In case of CD, surface passivation stabilizes the defect originated trap sites to facilitate the effective radiative recombination of trapped electron-hole pairs which is evident by the bright PL emission. The concept of radiative recombination in many ways found similar to the traditional quantum dots [378]. Several studies have justified the tunability and bright PL emission based on radiative recombination between the trap carriers such as electrons and holes localized within a small sp^2 carbon core and sp^3 defect hybrid matrix [379–381].

1.5. CD-based bacterial detection

Recently, CDs have been used for sensing biomolecules such as antibodies and aptamers for bio-imaging and sensitive detection of bacteria. This section presents different strategies employed to develop optical and electrochemical sensors based on CD for bacterial detection.

1.5.1 CD-based optical sensors for the detection of *E. coli*

In recent times, CDs have been explored intuitively for bio-imaging applications of bacterial cells such as *E. coli* [382]. *E. coli* are rod-shaped Gram-negative bacteria with sizes ranging from 1 to 3 μm. The cell wall of *E. coli* consists of adhesive fimbriae, an outer membrane of lipopolysaccharides (LPS), a periplasmic space with a peptidoglycan layer, and an inner cytoplasmic membrane [383,384].

Liu and co-workers identified *E. coli* ATCC 25922 cells (10^8 CFU mL^{-1}) by tagging them with biocompatible and multicolour CD. This was synthesized using passivated polyethylene glycol (PEG$_{1500N}$) following a wet chemistry procedure in an economical setup. The tagged *E. coli* cells were imaged under a confocal microscope with different excitation filters. The synthesized CDs were efficiently tagging to the bacterial cells [385]. Another study by Tripathi et al. was carried out on tagging *E. coli* cells using multicolour variant of carbon dots synthesized from carbon soot ("diesel soot"). This was further deployed for imaging *E. coli* cells [386]. Modified synthesis strategies to develop amphiphilic CD for bacterial detection were explored by Nandi et al. [387]. The amphiphilic carbon dots were synthesized using 6-O-acylated fatty acid ester of D-glucose precursor followed by carbonization. The presence of a hydrocarbon chain on the surface of CD ensures higher lipophilic interaction with the cell membrane of bacteria resulting in efficient tagging of *E. coli* cells. The outcome of CD as an efficient fluorescent nanoprobe for bio-imaging was promising. Shi et al. prepared unique P-doped carbon dots using sucrose and phosphoric acid for bio-imaging *E. coli* cells [388]. Likewise, Dubey and co-workers hydrothermally synthesized fluorescent water-soluble CDs from soya nuggets under insufficient oxygen. The synthesized CD was successfully used for imaging *E. coli* cells [389]. Bhaisare et al. synthesized magnetic carbon dots (Mag-CD) wherein the synthesized iron oxide nanoparticles were treated with the mixture of acetic acid and chitosan. The detection of *E. coli* in both standard and spiked urine samples was achieved using Mag-CD. The detection limit was found to be 4×10^3 CFU mL^{-1} [390]. The advancement in single-molecule based bio-imaging of *E. coli* cells was achieved using carbon dots. Here, confocal microscopy was used to image carbon dots tagged *E. coli* and HeLa cells. Multicolour emission signals were captured under different excitation lasers such as 401 nm (blue), 488 nm (green), and 639 nm (red) [391].

The bioimaging application of carbon dots was explored using various precursors and surface modifications to achieve facile and excellent bacterial labeling efficiency [392–402]. Among the several modifications on the CD surface, bacteria-derived CDs were widely used to identify and assess the viability of bacteria such as *E. coli*. In addition, the bacteria-derived CDs could also differentiate between dead and viable microbes by analyzing the PL emission response from the tagged bacterial cells [403–409].

Heteroatomic doped CDs were synthesized comprehensively for bio-imaging and detection of bacterial cells using n-type dopants like nitrogen-doped carbon dots.

Zhang and his group have synthesized nitrogen-doped carbon dots with ultra-high fluorescence quantum yield using ethanolamine and Tris precursors. The CDs proved to be efficient for bio-labeling and were used for the imaging of *E. coli* [410]. Other n-type dopants, such as phosphorus and sulphur have also been used for bacterial cell imaging and detection [388,411]. Several strategies have been deployed to use co-doped CDs modified with n and p-type dopants to enhance fluorescence emission signals for facile cell imaging [412]. The dopants such as lanthanum has been effectively used to image and detect *E. coli* and mammalian cells [413].

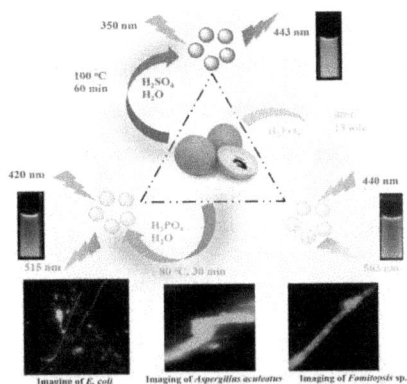

Fig. 1.13 Schematic procedure for the fabrication of blue-, green- and yellow- C-dots from Manilkara zapota fruits as a carbon source using H_2SO_4 and H_3PO_4 as oxidizing agents [421]

"Green" CDs have also been utilized to screen different bacterial species. Mehta and their group used *Saccharum officinarum* juice for the hydrothermal synthesis of water-soluble CDs. The bright fluorescent CD was screened for *E. coli* and yeast cell imaging applications [395]. Pal and co-workers adopted another simple green chemistry methodology wherein CD was synthesized from curcumin passivated with polyethyleneimine (PEI). These CDs were used for the detection of *E. coli* DH5-alpha and *S. aureus* [414]. The green synthesis of nitrogen-doped carbon dots was carried out from natural green pakchoi for demonstrating the bio-labeling property of CD against *E. coli* and HeLa cells [415]. The green synthesis was further explored by synthesizing CD from *Carica papaya* juice for bio-imaging *E. coli* and fungal cells [416]. Likewise, several natural precursors and carbon sources such as wheat straw

[417], papaya [418], gram shells [419], lemon and grapefruits [420], *Manilkara zapota* fruits [421] (Fig. 1.13) were used for the green synthesis of CD for *E. coli* tagging and cell imaging applications. In addition, a few green synthesized CDs reportedly possess antibacterial properties having strong peroxidase activity and reactive oxygen species for the lysing of bacterial cell walls [422–424].

The sensitive detection of *E. coli* cells was also achieved by functionalizing the surface of CD with carbohydrates such as mannose. The functionalized mannose selectively binds with the FimH lectin unit available on the surface of *E. coli* cells as shown in Fig. 1.14. The specificity induced due to mannose allowed the quantification of bacteria with a detection limit was 450 CFU mL^{-1}. This was also tested in real samples such as tap water, apple juice, and human urine [425]. In a similar kind of study, the group had synthesized mannose-CQD and folic acid-CQD to selectively detect *E. coli* and to induce the specific binding of CQD with folate receptors expressed in tumor cells [426].

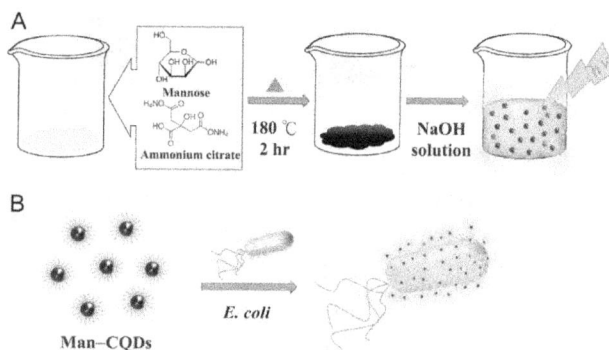

Fig.1.14 Schematic representations of (A) the synthesis of mannose-modified carbon quantum dots (Man–CQDs) from ammonium citrate and mannose and (B) their use in the selective labeling of E. coli [425]

Bhushan and co-workers presented a method where casein precursor was used for the hydrothermal synthesis of multicolour emissive carbon dots. The synthesized CDs were screened for the selective identification of *E. coli* over *S. aureus*. This selective exclusion is based on the electrostatic repulsion experienced between the anionic teichoic acid and negatively charged carbon dots [427]. The challenge of selective detection of *E. coli* was also addressed by re-engineering and passivating known antibiotics such as colistin and amikacin (Fig. 1.15) with the carbon dots [428,429].

Moreover, ethylenediamine-based CDs have also exhibited antimicrobial properties against bacteria such as *E. coli* synergistically with H_2O_2 [430]. Thus, CDs have emerged as potential antimicrobial agents and can be used effectively against antimicrobial-resistant bacteria [431,432].

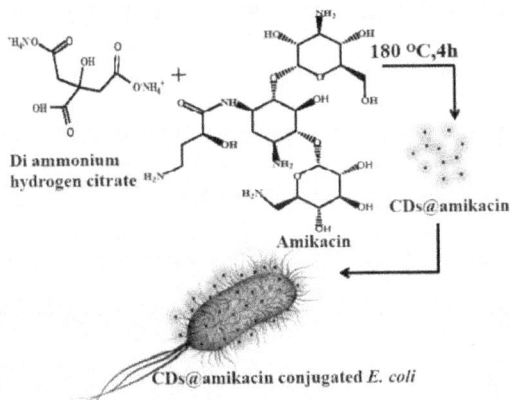

Fig. 1.15 Pictorial representation of amikacin passivated CD (CDs@amikacin) synthesis for specific detection of E. coli [428]

1.5.2 CD based electrochemical sensors for the detection of *E. coli*

Electrochemical sensors are a powerful tool for the sensitive and selective detection of bacteria such as *E. coli*. CD-based electrochemical sensors are not explored as much as CD-based optical sensors. In a very recent study, Pangajam et al. used conductive carbon dots/ZnO nanorod/PANI composite electrode as DNA biosensor for the sensitive detection of *E. coli* O157:H7 [433]. The presented electrochemical DNA biosensor exhibited a linear range from 1.3×10^{-18} M to 5.2×10^2 M with a detection limit of 1.3×10^{-18} M in water samples with selectivity towards *E. coli* O157:H7.

Another interesting study showed the fabrication of a wireless electrochemical device for bacteria detection using surface-coated electrochemically generated fluorescent carbon dots (FCDs) synthesized from cationic polymer as shown in Fig. 1.16. The FCD was integrated with cesium tungsten oxide ($CsWO_3$) to form a cationic nanohybrid. The interaction between the cationic $CsWO_3$ and anionic bacterial cell wall was investigated electrochemically. The LOD was determined to be < 10 CFU mL^{-1} for *E. coli* [434].

1.5.3 CD-based optical sensors for the detection of *S. aureus*

The bio-labeling application of carbon dots was also investigated on different bacterial species such as *S. aureus*. *S. aureus* is a round-shaped Gram-positive bacterium with a size range from 0.5 to 2 μm. The cell wall of *S. aureus* has 70% peptidoglycan, teichoic acid, and proteins [435–437]. The potential of CD as an efficient fluorescent probe was also screened by imaging and detecting *S. aureus* [438].

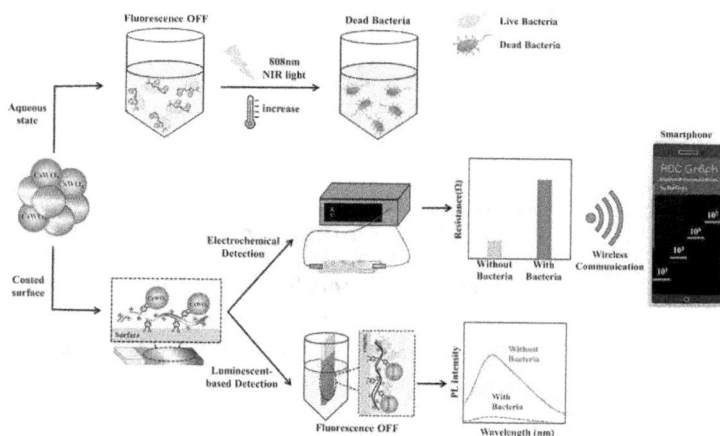

Fig. 1.16 Methodology for the wireless electrochemical set up for the detection of pathogenic bacteria based on $CsWO_3$ immobilized fluorescent carbon dots[434]

Mitra et al. synthesized a nanohybrid based on carbon nanoparticles and ZnO nanorod to determine bacterial cells such as *E. coli* and *S. aureus* [439]. The direct detection and cell imaging of *S. aureus* were achieved by surface passivation strategies. Nitrogen, phosphorus, sulphur, boron, and lanthanum doped carbon dots are also used for detecting bacteria such *S. aureus* [440–443]. A completely unique system based on hybrid CD-hydrogel was developed to detect Gram-positive bacteria

42

such as *B. anthracis* and *S. aureus*. The bacterial sensing within the hydrogel scaffold was based on the catalytic activity of bacterial enzymes, esterases and lipases, which acted on the ester bond within the hydrogel scaffold resulting in fluidization and quenching the fluorescence of CD [444]. The selective detection of *S. aureus* was achieved by modulating the surface properties of CD. The surface passivation of CD with quaternary ammonium compound is another strategy used to achieve selective detection of *S. aureus*. The well-known bactericidal activity of the quaternary ammonium compound, laurel betaine (BS-12), was explored by Yang and co-workers as shown in Fig. 1.17. The prepared quaternized BS-12 was successfully used for the selective detection of *S. aureus* and other Gram-positive bacteria. The insertion of quaternized BS-12 into the bacterial membrane was achieved using long hydrocarbon chain. These long alkyl chains induce the lipophilic interaction and easily pierce the peptidoglycan membrane of gram-positive bacteria. The cationic quaternary ammonium moiety in the close vicinity of the peptidoglycan layer exhibits strong attraction with the submerged anionic teichoic acid. This not only results in tagging of quaternized B-12 with the bacterial membrane but also ruptures the cell wall and act as antimicrobial agent. The synthesized CD was competent enough to tag multiple Gram-positive bacteria such as *S. aureus*, *M. luteus*, *B. subtilis* and could differentiate from Gram-negative bacteria [445].

Furthermore, a quaternary ammonium functionalized carbon dots using glycerol (carbon source), and dimethyloctadecyl[3-(trimethoxysilyl)propy]ammonium chloride (Si-QAC) was synthesized to detect Gram-positive bacteria selectively [446]. The fluorescent imaging of Gram-positive bacteria such as *S. aureus* reveals the selective nature of synthesized quaternary CD to induce contact-enhanced fluorescence emission after tagging bacterial cells (Fig. 1.18). On the other hand, there was no fluorescence emission from Gram-negative bacteria. This is due to the nature of the bacterial cell wall and its composition, as quaternary ammonium compounds exhibit affinity towards lipophilic molecules [447].

Similarly, Zhao et al. have successfully synthesized quaternary ammonium carbon compounds using 2,3-epoxypropyltrimethylammonium chloride and diallyldimethylammonium chloride by a facile "one-pot" method for the imaging of

43

Gram-positive bacteria. The antibacterial activity was confirmed with higher efficacy by analyzing the quantitative proteomics-based tandem mass tags.

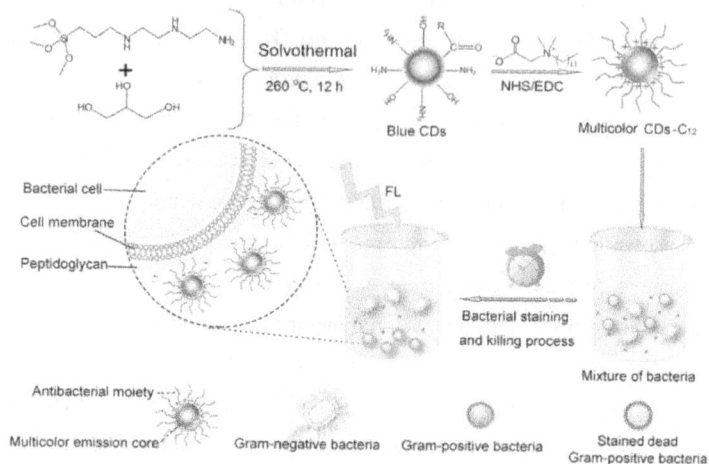

Fig. 1.17 Schematic illustrating the preparation of multicolour CDs-C$_{12}$ and their application in selective Gram-positive bacterial imaging and killing [445]

This study revealed that the quaternary ammonium compound must have intervened in the protein translational, post-translational modification, and protein turnover within bacterial cells [448].

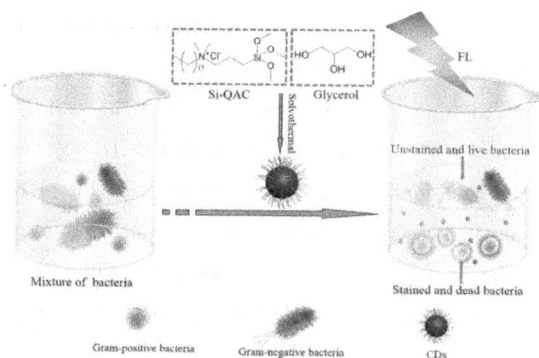

Fig. 1.18 Schematic illustrating the preparation of quaternized CDs and their application for selective imaging and killing of Gram-positive bacteria [448]

Yang et al. encapsulated CD in organosilane shells by cohydrolyzation of tetraethyl orthosilicate and bis[3-(triethoxysilyl)propyl] disulfide to form core–shell CDs. This was used to amplify the fluorescence signal for the detection of *S. aureus*. The sensitivity of the bacterial detection increased multiple folds when the nanocapsules were coupled with immunological recognition and magnetic separation. The sensitivity of the developed system was 108 times more than that of conventional immunoassays labeled with carbon dots [449].

CD has also been re-engineered by passivating its surface with known antibiotics such as vancomycin. It is a broad spectrum of glycopeptide antibiotics with a higher effectivity against bacteria like *S. aureus* and MRSA (methicillin resistant *Staphylococcus aureus*) and is clinically relevant to treat infections. Zhong et al. exploited the selectivity of vancomycin towards *S. aureus* by forming a hydrogen bond with D-ala-D-ala repeating subunits of amino acids available at the peptidoglycan membrane. The vancomycin passivated CD could detect *S. aureus* with a linear range of $3.18 \times 10^5 - 1.59 \times 10^8$ CFU mL^{-1} with a detection limit of 9.40×10^4 CFU mL^{-1} [450].

1.5.4 CD-based electrochemical sensors for the detection of *S. aureus*

As mentioned in section 1.5.2, the FCD integrated cesium tungsten oxide (CsWO$_3$) cationic nanohybrid-based electrochemical sensor was also used for the detection of *S. aureus* with a detection limit of <10 CFU mL^{-1} [434].

1.5.5 CD-based optical & electrochemical sensors for the detection of different pathogenic bacteria

The CD and related carbon nanomaterials have also been used for the detection of different pathogenic bacteria such as *Salmonella*, *Pseudomonas*, and *Mycobacterium tuberculosis*.

Salmonella is a rod-shaped Gram-negative flagellated bacterium [451]. A unique strategy for detecting *Salmonella* using red and blue fluorescent magnetite CD (CD-Fe$_3$O$_4$) nanoparticle composite was developed by Paramanik and co-workers. The developed optical sensor specifically detects *Salmonella* and distinguishes it from MRSA in blood samples by multicolour fluorescent cell imaging. *Salmonella* was detected selectively by AMP attached with magnetic CD, and the magnetic nature of CD was exploited for the separation and enrichment for diagnosis [452]. Similarly, aptamer conjugated carbon dot was utilized by Wang and the group for the quick and sensitive detection of *Salmonella* with a lower detection limit of 50 CFU mL^{-1}. The efficiency of the developed probe was tested in real samples such as egg samples and tap water [453]. Likewise, *Salmonella* detection was carried out in food samples to prevent a threat to animal and human health [454].

The detection of *Pseudomonas aeruginosa* was also carried out in many studies using carbon dots and carbon nanomaterials. *P. aeruginosa* is a rod-shaped Gram-negative pathogenic bacterium, typically present in hospital settings and prevails as a major source of nosocomial infections [455,456]. In a recent study, Ahmadian et al. designed a nanocomposite wherein the carbon nano template was synthesized from soot followed by modifications using NiFe$_2$O$_4$ nanoparticles. The novel nanostructure was used to detect *P. aeruginosa* by measuring the fluorescence emission from the tagged bacterial cells [456]. The selective detection of *P. aeruginosa* was achieved by Otis et al. by synthesizing carbon dots using aminoguanidine and citric acid precursors. The aminoguanidine residues on the CDs' contributed to the selective detection and antibacterial activity against *P. aeruginosa* [457].

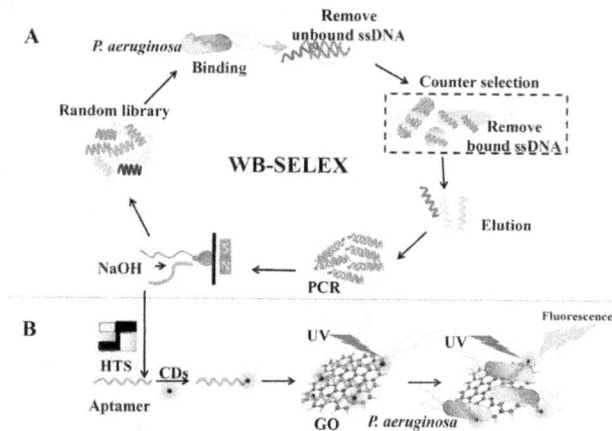

Fig. 1.19 A pictorial representation for the development of the fluorescence assay to detect P. aeruginosa based on aptamer/CD/graphene conjugate [458]

Furthermore, a culture-independent detection of *P. aeruginosa* was developed by Wang et al. The developed system consisted of highly specific aptamers conjugated with carbon dots (fluorescence probe) and graphene (quencher). The graphene anchor aptamer (π–π stacking) and graphene's quenching ability could substantially remove the background fluorescence, resulting in enhanced detection sensitivity. Aptamer-CD probe/GO system was used for the sensitive and selective detection of *P. aeruginosa* [458] as shown in Fig. 1.19. The carbon dots have also been used for tagging the extracellular polymeric substances (EPS) scaffold of *P. aeruginosa*. The results confirmed the significant dendritic morphology of *P. aeruginosa* EPS with the help of fluorescence microscopy [459]. The biofilm imaging of different micro-organisms, including *P. aeruginosa* was also achieved using CD [392].

Mycobacterium is highly virulent and causes tuberculosis through one of its strains (*M. tuberculosis*) with a higher mortality rate. The mycobacterial cell wall is composed of a peptidoglycan layer, mycolic acid (MA), and arabinogalactan (AG). The cell wall of mycobacterium strikes resemblance with Gram-positive and Gram-negative cell envelopes [460]. As a part of optical detection, CDs have been deployed for the detection of mycobacterium. The hydrothermally synthesized CDs have been used as a direct tagging probe for the detection of *M. tuberculosis, P. aeruginosa,* and *M. oryzae* cells [461].

1.6 Research Gap

The antimicrobial-resistant bacteria have been evolving against several antibiotics with time and become life-threatening in no time. There is a clear requirement in establishing the research need and efforts across the globe to deal with this challenge. A few knowledge gaps have been identified, which demand immediate research, i. rapid and robust identification of Gram-negative and Gram-positive bacteria, ii. a non-toxic and biocompatible probe for screening bacterial cells, iii. sensitive and selective detection of bacteria in polymicrobial and real samples, and iv. feasibility of the bacteria detection method to make it affordable and user-friendly with socio-economic impact.

1.7 Motivation

The existing bacterial detection methods have been used for several decades with inevitable limitations. The drawbacks are not only restricted to time consumption, low throughput, portability, sensitivity, and selectivity, but it demands the availability of skilled labor. Although bacterial detection has been improved with technological advancements, these attempts have not been sufficient to overcome the drawbacks. Recently, the nanomaterials like carbon dots have emerged as a suitable option for simple, rapid, sensitive, and selective detection of bacteria. The development of novel carbon dots-based fluorimetric and impedimetric sensors has motivated the sensitive and selective detection of pathogenic bacteria.

1.8 Novelty

Recently, the rise of antimicrobial-resistant bacteria has become a point of concern due to the mortality rate and non-availability of proper and effective treatment. This can be overcome by rapid and accurate sensing of pathogenic bacteria, which may curb the overuse of antibiotics. The development of a sensing system is essential for detecting and controlling the bacteria causing life-threatening diseases such as sepsis, tuberculosis, and food/waterborne illness. The traditional diagnostic assays involve time-consuming methods, complicated procedures, and expensive laboratory settings. With the emergence of nanotechnology, bacterial testing has been revolutionized dramatically. The various types of nanomaterials, such as carbon dots, have intrinsic optical and electronic properties that can be used to develop bacterial biosensors. The carbon dots-based optical (fluorimetric) and electrochemical (impedimetric) sensors will revamp the monitoring of lethal pathogenic bacteria with high throughput screening and affordable technology.

To the best of our knowledge, presented novel heteroatomic doped carbon dots were never introduced as fluorimetric and impedimetric sensors to detect multiple pathogenic bacteria. Several variants of N and N/ S doped carbon dots have been used to bio-image different bacteria. Also, the unique pH-sensitive carbon dots were synthesized for the cell imaging and detection of Gram-negative and Gram-positive bacteria. The novel colistin passivated carbon dots synthesized from citric acid and ethylenediamine have never been used for the selective sensing of Gram-negative bacteria in standard, real and polymicrobial samples. The unique colistin carbon dots immobilized within agarose matrix over disposable screen-printed carbon electrodes have never been reported to detect Gram-negative bacteria in real and polymicrobial samples, which further enhances the novelty of the presented work.

1.9 Objectives and scope of the work

The main objective of the present work is to develop fluorimetric and impedimetric sensors for the selective detection of pathogenic bacteria using carbon dots. Fluorescent imaging and sensing of bacterial cells were performed using N-doped and N/S- co-doped CDs. The surface passivated CD was also used to probe specific bacteria in polymicrobial samples. The enhanced electronic properties of CDs coupled with the selectivity of colistin towards Gram-negative bacteria were utilized to develop a novel, label-free, disposable impedimetric sensor for the detection of *E. coli* in real and clinical samples.

The scope of this work includes:

- Microwave-assisted and hydrothermal synthesis of novel N-doped, N/S co-doped, and colistin passivated carbon dots and their characterization.

- Fluorescence cell imaging of pathogenic bacteria using the N/S co-doped carbon dots.

- pH-dependent imaging and sensing of pathogenic bacteria using N-doped carbon dots.

- Selective fluorescence detection of Gram-negative bacteria using colistin passivated carbon dots.

- Label-free impedimetric sensing of Gram-negative bacteria using colistin modified screen-printed carbon electrode (SPCE).

- Testing and validation of developed sensors with real and clinical samples.

Chapter 2

Materials and methods

2. Materials and methods

The details of various chemicals and reagents used for the synthesis of carbon dots, instruments used for the characterization, protocols for tagging, imaging, and quantifying the pathogenic bacteria are discussed in this chapter. The procedures which are not common for all the chapters are presented at the beginning of each chapter.

2.1 Chemicals and reagents

Tris(hydroxymethyl)aminomethane, thiourea, citric acid, glycine, cysteamine, colistin, and MTT assay kit were purchased from Sigma-Aldrich (USA). Ethylenediamine (EDA), ethylenediaminetetraacetic acid (EDTA), and glacial acetic acid were of analytical grade and used without further purification. The media preparation for growing bacterial culture was carried out using peptone, yeast extract, and sodium chloride procured from Hi-media Pvt. Ltd. (India). The readymade media (Difco™ LB Broth and LB Agar) were procured from BD (USA) for bacterial culturing. Biomedical grade carbon, silver, and silver chloride conducting paste, along with their solvents, were purchased from DuPont (USA). All the other chemicals used for the study were of analytical grade and used as received. Milli-Q water (18.2 MΩ cm) was used to prepare solutions throughout the study.

2.2 Instrumentation

The absorption spectrum was recorded using a UV-1700 Pharmaspec spectrophotometer, Shimadzu (Japan). Fourier transform infra red (FTIR) spectrum was scanned using Thermo Nicolet, and Bruker (USA) spectrophotometers. PL emission measurements were carried out using Cary Eclipse Fluorescence Spectrophotometer, Agilent (USA). X-Ray photoelectron spectroscopy (XPS) analysis was performed using an Axis-Ultra, Shimadzu (Kratos Analytical Ltd., UK). Different electrochemical techniques were carried out using electrochemical analyzer CHI608D (CH Instruments, USA). The morphological analysis was performed using a high-resolution transmission electron microscope (HRTEM) (JEM-2100, JEOL (Japan)), atomic force microscopy (AFM) ((Park systems- XE70, (Seoul, South Korea)) and a field emission scanning electron microscope (FESEM), Carl Zeiss (Germany). The X-ray diffraction (XRD) analysis was carried out with Miniflex 600 diffractometer, Rigaku Corporation (USA). The zeta potential analysis and DLS particle size measurement was performed using Particle Analyzer (Litesizer 500, Anton Paar, Austria) and Malver Zetasizer (UK). The fluorescence microscopic images were acquired using Axio Vert. A1, Carl Zeiss (Germany). MTT assay was carried out using a multiwell plate reader Synergy HT, BioTek (USA). The carbon dots were synthesized using a domestic microwave oven, IFB-20PG4S (India). The pH measurements were carried using a pH meter, Hanna instruments (USA).

2.3 Preparation of phosphate buffer saline

The composition of the phosphate-buffered saline (0.1 M) with pH 7.4 used in this work is shown in Table 2.1.

Table 2.1 Composition of 0.1 M PBS (pH 7.4)

Sl. No.	Chemicals	Amount (g L^{-1})
1	Sodium chloride	80.0
2	Potassium chloride	2.0
3	Disodium hydrogen phosphate	14.4
4	Potassium dihydrogen phosphate	2.4

2.4 Quantum yield estimation

The quantum yield of carbon dots was estimated using equation 2.1 with quinine sulfate in 0.1 M H_2SO_4 (quantum yield, 54%) as the standard [373,410].

$$\Phi_{sample} = \frac{Ab_{std}}{Ab_{sample}} \times \frac{PL_{sample}}{PL_{std}} \times \frac{m^2_{sample}}{m^2_{std}} \times \Phi_{std} \tag{2.1}$$

where, Φ_{sample} and Φ_{std} are the photoluminiscent quantum yield (PLQY) of the test and standard samples, respectively; PL_{sample} and PL_{std} refer to the PL emission intensity of the sample and the standard compound in the emission region from 400 to 600 nm; Ab_{sample} and Ab_{std} are the absorbance of the test and the standard samples, and m^2_{sample} and m^2_{std} are the refractive indices of test and standard (water is taken as the solvent for the test sample and sulfuric acid for the standard).

2.5 Bacterial cell cultivation assay

The different bacterial strains such as *Escherichia coli, Staphylococcus aureus, Proteus vulgaris, Pseudomonas aeruginosa, Bacillus subtilis,* and *Mycobacterium smegmatis* were opted for the experimental investigations. The laboratory glassware used for bacteria cell culture was sterilized in an autoclave with standard procedures and conditions. The Luria-Bertani (LB) media (peptone, yeast extract, and sodium chloride prepared in MilliQ water) was sterilized and used as a nutrient source to grow bacteria in a sterile environment. A single colony of each bacterial strain was inoculated in sterilized LB broth (5 mL) overnight in a shaker – incubator at 37 °C, 180 rpm. The growth of the bacterial culture was monitored at 600 nm (OD_{600}). The bacterial cells were pelleted at 5500 rpm for 10 minutes and washed with MilliQ water or PBS. The washed cells were finally reconstituted and used for tagging with CD.

2.6 Cytotoxicity assay

The cytotoxicity of the prepared carbon dots was evaluated by MTT (3-(4,5-dimethylthiazol-2-yl)-2,5-diphenyltetrazolium bromide) assay [462]. In brief, 10^8 CFU mL^{-1} bacterial cells were incubated with different concentrations of CD for 24 hours. From the incubated sample, 100 µL was aliquot into a multiwell plate followed by adding 10 µL MTT (5 mg mL^{-1}) to each well. It was then incubated for 4 hours at 37 °C. The medium was then carefully aspirated, and 100 µL of solubilization solution was added to each well to dissolve the formed formazan crystals. After 15 minutes of incubation on a rotary shaker, the optical density of each well was measured at 690 nm to obtain the background readings of the solution and at 570 nm to get the actual readings from the sample. The percentage viability was calculated using Equation 2.2:

$$\% viability = \frac{(OD_{sample} - OD_{blank})}{(OD_{control} - OD_{blank})} \times 100 \tag{2.2}$$

where, OD_{sample} and $OD_{control}$ are the optical density of bacterial cells treated with and without carbon dots, respectively, at 570 nm, and OD_{blank} is the optical density of background at 690 nm.

2.7 Fluorescence microscopic studies on CD tagged bacterial cells and human buccal epithelial cells (hBEC)

The bacterial cells were washed to remove media, mixed with various concentrations of CD, and incubated for 60 minutes at room temperature. After incubation, the CD-tagged cells were washed twice to remove the unbound CD. After washing, the CD-tagged bacterial cells were imaged using a fluorescence microscope. Similarly, the tagging potential of CD was investigated on the hBEC. The saliva was diluted using 0.1 M PBS to reduce the viscosity of the sample, followed by centrifugation at 2000 rpm for 5 minutes. The salivary cell pellet was dissolved in 0.1 M PBS. The hBEC and CD were mixed in an equal volume ratio followed by incubation for 60 minutes at RT. After incubation and washing, the CD tagged hBEC was imaged under a fluorescence microscope with different excitation filters at 40X magnification. The corresponding blue, green and red emission was obtained from the tagged cells when imaged under corresponding excitation filters.

2.8 Fluorescence spectroscopy studies of the CD tagged bacterial cells

Fluorescence spectrophotometric analysis was carried out to study the photoluminescence (PL) emission response obtained from CD-tagged bacterial cells. The cells were grown overnight in LB media at 37 °C and 180 rpm in a shaker incubator. The bacterial culture was centrifuged at 5500 rpm for 10 minutes to pellet down the cells. The cell pellet was washed twice with PBS. The washed cells were mixed gently with CD solution and incubated at 37 °C for 2 hours. After incubation, the cells were washed thrice in MilliQ water to remove the unbound CD. The PL intensity of CD-tagged bacteria cells was measured at various excitation wavelengths.

2.9 Calculation of limit of detection (LOD)

The LOD was calculated for the fluorimetric and impedimetric sensors using the reported procedure [463]. The expression for LOD is,

$$LOD = \frac{3 \times standard\ deviation}{slope\ of\ linear\ regression} \tag{2.3}$$

Minimum 10 replicate measurements were performed in the blank solution to obtain the precise LOD values. Finally, the obtained slope of the calibration plot was used along with standard deviation to calculate the detection limit.

Chapter 3

Synthesis of different multi-emissive N/S co-doped carbon dots for the detection of pathogenic bacteria

3. Synthesis of different multi-emissive N/S co-doped carbon dots for the detection of pathogenic bacteria

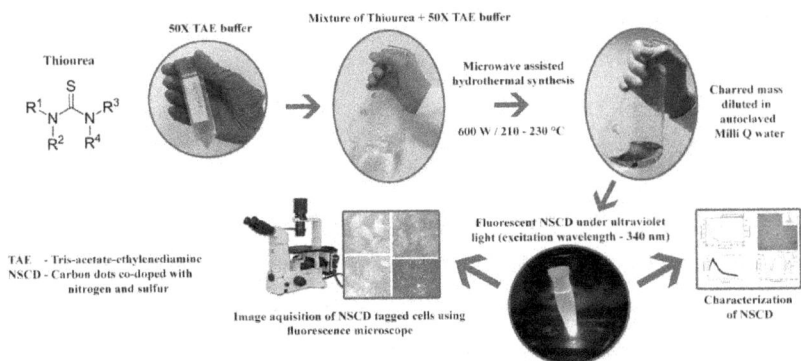

This chapter explains the synthesis of novel nitrogen/sulphur (N/S) co-doped carbon dots with brilliant bacterial tagging efficiency. The microwave synthesis of N/S co-doped carbon dots has been carried out by deploying different precursors combinations such as thiourea/50X TAE buffer (NSCD) and cysteamine/50X TAE buffer (Cy@CD). Both the variants of N/S co-doped carbon dots were characterized to investigate their spectral, morphological, and chemical composition. N/S co-doped carbon dots were used as nanoprobes to detect different bacteria such as *Escherichia coli*, *Staphylococcus aureus*, *Klebsiella pneumoniae* and *Pseudomonas aeruginosa* and mammalian cells such as human buccal epithelial cells (hBEC). The one-step facile synthesis of N/S co-doped carbon dots provides cost-effective and ready-to-use nanomaterial with excellent optical sensor characteristics for cell imaging applications.

3.1 Experimental methodology

3.1.1 Microwave synthesis of NSCD

The one-step microwave-assisted synthesis was carried out using thiourea and 50X TAE buffer as a novel precursor combination in a 2:5 (w/v) ratio. The simple one-step synthesis of carbon dots was conducted in a domestic microwave oven at 800 W for 15 minutes. As the reaction completed, the temperature of the microwave was allowed to drop at room temperature (RT). The charred mass was dissolved in 15 mL of autoclaved ultra-pure MilliQ water followed by sonication for 10 minutes. The stock solution of CD was centrifuged at 14000 rpm for 60 minutes to remove the unreacted impurities of carbon dots. CD was then purified using a 0.2 micron syringe filter followed by overnight dialysis using a 1 kDa dialysis membrane. Finally, CD solution was diluted to a pale yellow colour solution (0.1 mg mL^{-1}) for performing further assays.

3.1.2 Microwave synthesis of Cy@CD

A similar methodology was applied for the synthesis of Cy@CD using cysteamine/50X TAE buffer precursor combination in a 2:5 (w/v) ratio. After allowing the temperature to drop slowly at room temperature, the brown colour charred mass was dissolved in 10 mL of autoclaved ultra-pure MilliQ water followed by sonication for 10 minutes. The dissolved Cy@CD solution was centrifuged at 12000 rpm for 60 minutes to remove the unreacted impurities of carbon dots. The purification of Cy@CD solution was carried out using a 0.22 micron syringe filter and overnight dialysis using a 1 kDa dialysis membrane. The stock concentration of Cy@CD was found to be 1.35 mg mL^{-1} and was diluted to a specific working concentration (2.25 µg mL^{-1}) for further studies.

3.2 Results and discussion

3.2.1 Spectroscopic characterization

The optical properties of water-soluble NSCD were probed at room temperature. Under bright light, the aqueous solution was yellow, but under a long-wavelength UV lamp, the solution colour changed to bright blue. The UV-Vis absorption spectrum (as shown in Fig. 3.1A) projected two distinct peaks. The absorption peak at 260 nm wavelength was attributed to $\pi \rightarrow \pi^*$ transition of aromatic sp^2 domain with damper PL emission. The weak absorption peak at 330 nm wavelength is predominantly due to the n$\rightarrow \pi^*$ transition of the C=O bond or C=N bond and elucidate the genesis of carbon dots.

Moreover, the high-intensity PL emission peak of NSCD was observed, and the fluorescent property of NSCD was demonstrated. The PL emission behavior was investigated at different excitation wavelengths, as shown in Fig. 3.1B. The PL emission peak shifted to a shorter wavelength (blueshift) when the excitation

56

wavelength was 270 to 300 nm. This may be because of un-reacted 50X TAE, which did not participate in NSCD synthesis. When the excitation wavelength varies from 300 to 340 nm, the corresponding PL emission shifts towards a longer wavelength (redshift). As a result, the fluorescence emission becomes intense, reaches a maximum at 340 nm excitation, and the PL emission was observed at 426 nm. The further change in excitation wavelength from 350 to 500 nm also showed a shift in PL emission towards a longer wavelength. But fluorescence intensity reduced and became weaker. Therefore after analyzing the PL emission spectra, the excitation wavelength-dependent PL emission behavior has been established.

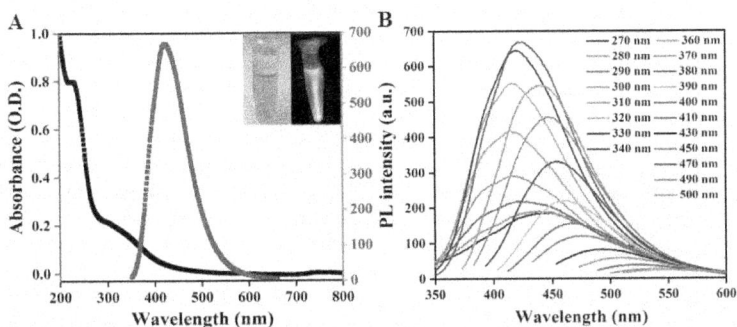

Fig. 3.1 A) UV-Vis absorption spectrum of NSCD (black) and PL emission curve at 360 nm excitation wavelength (blue). (Inset- Day-light and fluorescence images of NSCD) B) PL emission spectra of NSCD at the different excitation wavelength (270-500 nm)

The characterization of spectral properties of Cy@CD was also carried out using UV-Vis absorption and PL emission spectroscopy. The UV-Vis absorption spectrum (Fig. 3.2A) shows a typical intense peak at 230 nm and a feeble peak at 350 nm. This attributes to $\pi-\pi^*$ transition of aromatic sp^2 carbon domain (C=C) and $n-\pi^*$ transition due to C=O and nitrogen lone pair of electrons available on the surface Cy@CD [464].

The Cy@CD solution shows transparent pale yellow in daylight and bright blue under UV lamp. A strong PL emission was exhibited at 434 nm corresponding to 350 nm excitation. The intriguing excitation-dependent emission property of carbon dots was also observed for Cy@CD during the emission scan at the different excitation wavelengths (Fig. 3.2B). As the excitation wavelength changes from 300 to 350 nm, the emission intensity increases to the maximum with a redshift. The further change in excitation wavelength from 360 to 500 nm exhibited a dramatic reduction in the PL emission intensity with a perceptible redshift. The excitation-dependent emission behaviour of Cy@CD could be due to quantum confinement or the presence of surface defects [465].

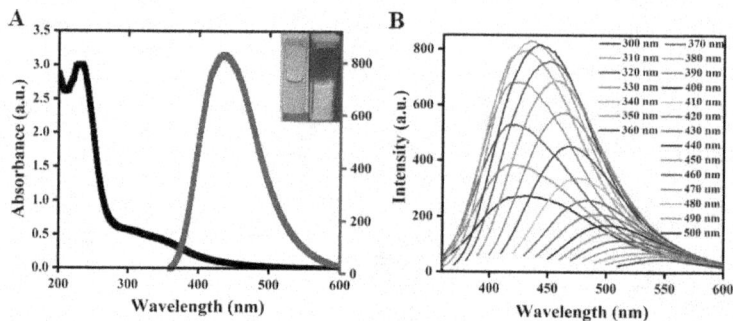

Fig. 3.2 A) UV-Vis absorption spectrum of Cy@CD (black) and PL emission curve at 360 nm excitation wavelength (blue). (Inset- Day-light and fluorescence images of Cy@CD) B) PL emission spectra of NSCD at the different excitation wavelength (300-500 nm)

3.2.2 Morphological characterization

High-Resolution Transmission Electron Microscopy (HR-TEM) micrograph of NSCD (Fig. 3.3A) shows almost uniform and well separated spherical particles. The size variations reside in the range of 1.65 to 6.7 nm. The histogram plot exhibited the average diameter of forty NSCD particles and was measured as 3.6 ± 0.88 nm (Fig. 3.3B). The XRD pattern of NSCD (Fig. 3.3C) shows a broad diffraction peak centered at $2\theta = 19.5°$, which is attributed to the turbostratic graphitic carbon phase.

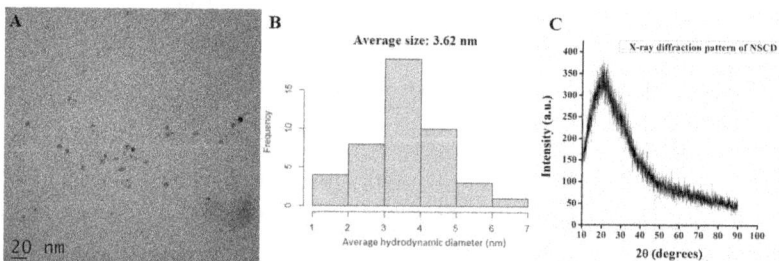

Fig. 3.3 A) HR-TEM images of NSCD to analyze the surface morphology and B) the average hydrodynamic diameter was found to be 3.6 ± 0.88 nm. (Scale bar- 20 nm) C) X-ray diffraction pattern of NSCD.

58

The morphology of Cy@CD was also analyzed by HR-TEM to determine its shape and size. Fig. 3.4A shows uniformly spherical Cy@CD particles with slender size distribution. The average diameter of fifty Cy@CD particles was calculated as 3.38 ± 0.9 nm (Fig. 3.4B). The inset in Fig. 3.4A shows the well-resolved lattice fringes with measured d-spacing to be 0.24 nm. This attributes to the graphitic lattice plane (1 0 0) and therefore suggests that CDs possess a graphitic structure.

XRD analysis of Cy@CD (Fig. 3.4C) revealed the broad diffraction peak due to the small size Cy@CD and is analogous to the peak of graphitic carbon with $2\theta = 20.97°$. Dynamic Light Scattering (DLS) measurement of Cy@CD revealed the average hydrodynamic diameter. The measured size (5.26 nm) was slightly bigger than the size of TEM analysis as shown in Fig. 3.4D.

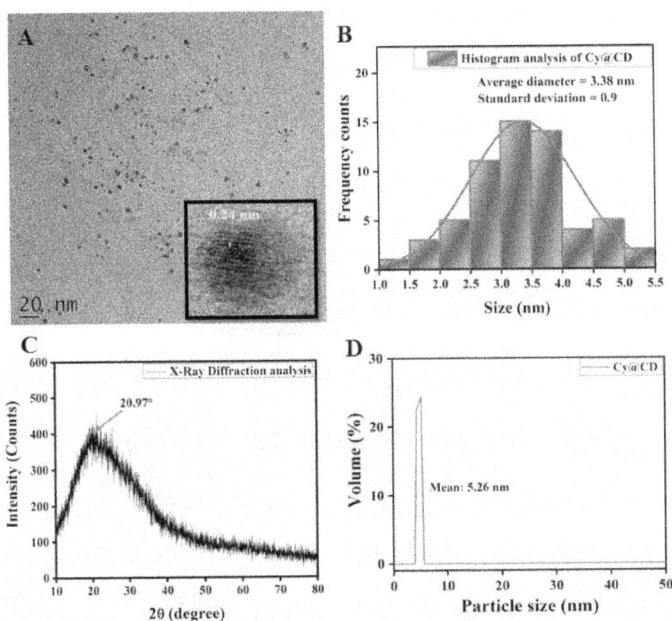

Fig. 3.4 A) HR-TEM micrograph of Cy@CD (Inset: shows the lattice fringes), B) Histogram plot for narrow size distribution of Cy@CD particles, C) XRD analysis & D) DLS analysis of Cy@CD exhibiting the average hydrodynamic diameter

3.2.3 Chemical composition analysis

Fourier transform infrared (FTIR) spectrum of the NSCD is shown in Fig. 3.5A. The typical absorption band at 3354.12 cm^{-1} is due to the stretching vibrations of O-H (alcohol), which provides information on the hydrophilic nature of newly synthesized NSCD. The peak at 2937.73 cm^{-1} significantly determines the presence of stretching vibrations of C-H. The peak at 1650 cm^{-1} is attributed to the stretching vibrations of C=O. The absorption band at 1462.75 cm^{-1} is ascribed to the bending vibrations of C-H. The band range from 1000 to 1300 cm^{-1} is assigned to the C=C, C=S, C-O and C-N functional groups on the NSCD. The FTIR results showed the availability of hydrophilic groups on the surface of NSCD to validate its excellent water solubility and stability in the aqueous system. The chemical composition and chemical bonds of NSCD were further investigated by deploying X-Ray PS. The wide spectrum scan (Fig. 3.5B) result stipulates that NSCD are comprised of carbon (C 1s), oxygen (O 1s), nitrogen (N 1s), and sulfur (S 2p). The atomic percentage is 72.60% for C 1s (maximum), 17.79% for O 1s, 9.20% for N 1s, and 2.41% for S 2p, respectively.

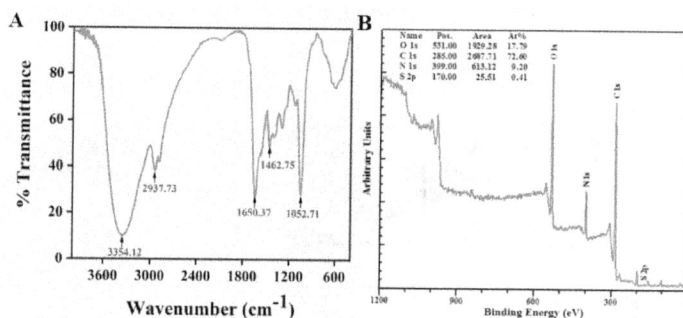

Fig. 3.5 A) FTIR spectra for functional group analysis present on the surface of NSCD B) XPS wide scan spectrum to analyze the chemical composition of NSCD

The results of FT-IR and XPS showed excellent consistency with each other. Hence, the presence of N and S dopants on the surface of NSCD was confirmed. XPS de-convoluted elemental spectra have been shown in Fig. 3.6. The high-resolution XPS spectrum of C 1s was de-convoluted to four peaks with binding energies at 284.1 eV for C-C, C=C and C-S, 285.60 eV for C-O, C-N and C-O-C, 287.01 eV for C-OH and C=O and 288.23 eV for O-C=O. The high-resolution spectrum for O 1s shows two peaks at 531.88 eV and 533 eV assigned to organic C-O and C=O. The S 2p high-resolution spectrum was de-convoluted to two peaks only at binding energy 165.24 and 167.75 eV and was attributed to organosulphur (C-S) and oxidized sulfate C-SOx (x = 2, 3, 4) species. The high-resolution spectrum of N 1s was de-convoluted to two peaks at binding energy 399 and 401.21 eV and ascribed to pyridinic and pyrrolic N.

The chemical composition of NSCD deciphers its stability due to the charged functional groups. The various functional groups such as carboxylic, hydroxyl and carbonyl are responsible in providing similar charges on NSCD. These charged functional groups on the particles leads to the electrostatic repulsion and prevent them from aggregation. Therefore, the newly synthesized NSCD is relatively stable and does not show any dynamic behavior.

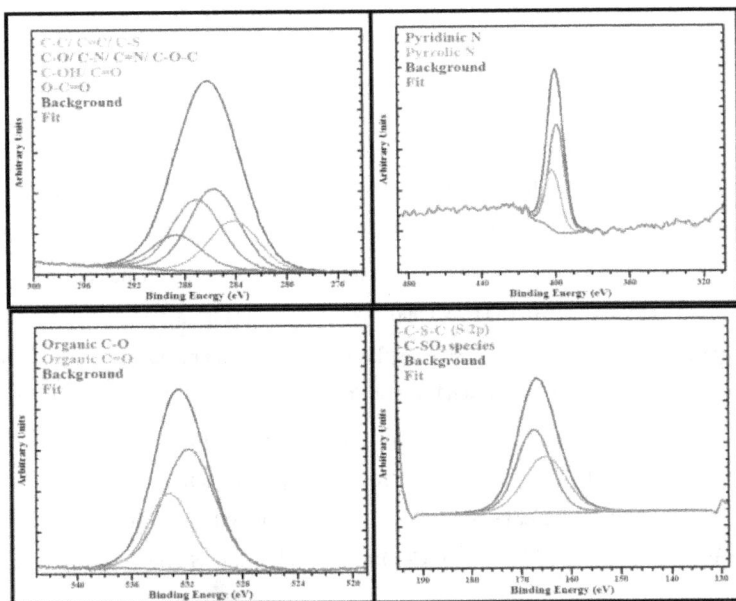

Fig. 3.6 De-convoluted spectra of XPS for carbon, oxygen, nitrogen and sulfur to analyze the chemical composition present on the surface of as-prepared NSCD

FTIR spectroscopy of Cy@CD (Fig. 3.7) revealed the functional groups available on the surface of synthesized carbon dots. The sharp peak at 3340 cm^{-1} ascribed to the presence of primary amine (-NH$_2$). The dual peak at 2940 cm^{-1} corresponds to the presence of an alkane functional group. The peak at 1630 cm^{-1} attributes to the N-H bending. The sharper peak at 1014 cm^{-1} corresponds to the presence of the organosulphur group (C-S).

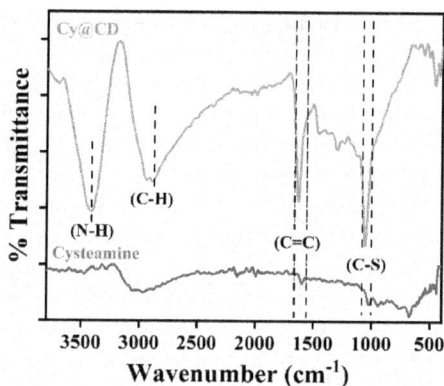

Fig. 3.7 FTIR spectra of Cy@CD and Cysteamine

The presence of the amine and organosulphur groups confirms the presence of nitrogen and sulphur dopants on the surface of Cy@CD. XPS analysis was carried out (Fig. 3.8) to confirm the composition of N, S, C, and O elements. The wide scan spectrum of Cy@CD showed the presence of four typical peaks of C 1s (285 eV), N 1s (400 eV), O 1s (531 eV) and S 2p (167 eV) (Fig. 3.8A). The de-convoluted XPS spectrum of C 1s (Fig. 3.8B) displayed two prominent peaks at 284.8 and 285.8 eV attributing to C=C and C-OH or C-O functional groups. The high-resolution spectrum of N 1s (Fig. 3.8C) de-convoluted in three relevant peaks at 398.1, 399.5, 401.3 eV, corresponding to pyridinic nitrogen, primary amine, and pyrrolic nitrogen, respectively. Fig. 3.8D showed O 1s de-convoluted spectrum exhibited the presence of single peak at 531.1 eV for C=O functional group. S 2p high-resolution spectrum

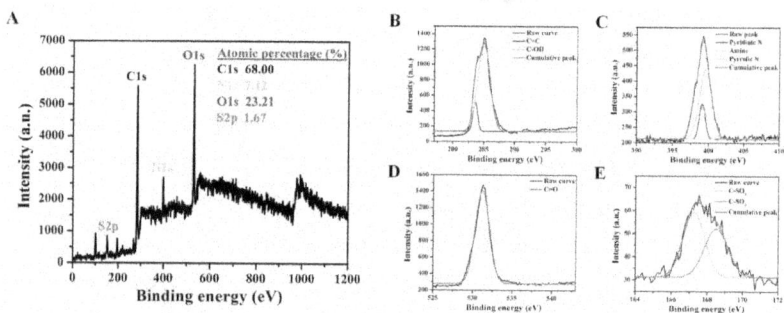

Fig. 3.8 A) Wide scan spectrum of Cy@CD, and B) high-resolution XPS spectra of C 1s, C) N 1s, D) O 1s and E) S 2p

confirms the presence of two peaks at 167.2 and 168.4 eV, which confirms the presence of organosulphur group (C-SOx- where x= 2, 3, 4) as shown in Fig. 3.8E. The XPS analysis of Cy@CD exhibited the successful doping of nitrogen and sulphur within the matrix of Cy@CD. The results obtained from XPS spectra are in close agreement with the FTIR results.

3.2.4 Stability of Cy@CD at different conditions

The stability of the fluorescent carbon dots was analyzed under different ionic concentrations, temperature, time interval, and pH. In brief, 5 µL of Cy@CD is mixed with different concentrations of NaCl, and fluorescent intensity was measured at an excitation wavelength of 350 nm. With an increase in ionic concentration from 0.1 to 1 M, there was no significant increase in the fluorescent intensity of the carbon dots (Fig. 3.9A). The Cy@CD solutions were prepared (2.25 µg mL^{-1}) and incubated under continuous UV-irradiation, and PL intensity was measured at a different time interval. No substantial decay was observed in PL intensity under different UV-irradiation times, as shown in Fig. 3.9C. Likewise, a similar concentration of Cy@CD solution was prepared and incubated at a different temperature like 4, 25, 50, 80 °C

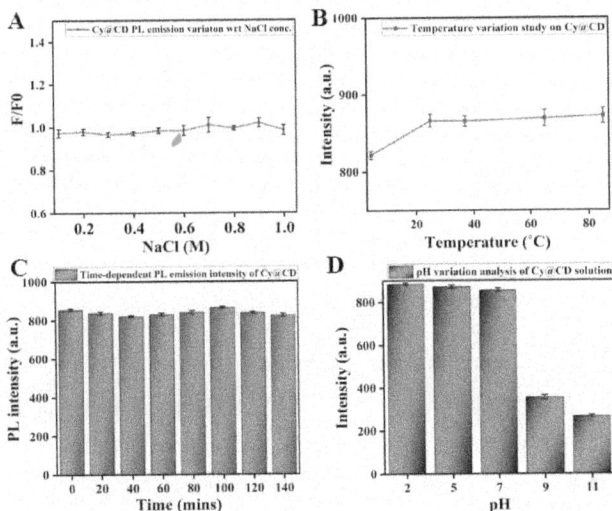

Fig. 3.9 A) PL emission response of Cy@CD at A) various NaCl concentration, B) different temperature, C) different UV irradiation time, and D) different pH

63

for 24 hours. The PL intensity was consistent for temperatures other than 4 °C (Fig. 3.9B). Therefore, the results obtained after screening the PL emission response of Cy@CD at different parameters such as ionic concentration, temperature, and time exhibited brilliant stability.

The pH of the Cy@CD stock solution was found to be 7. The pH of Cy@CD solution was adjusted to 2, 5, 9 and 11 by using standard 1 M HCl and NaOH solution to examine the pH-based variations in PL emission. The PL emission of Cy@CD showed a stable response from pH 2 to 7 (Fig. 3.9D). There was a substantial decay in fluorescence emission intensity at alkaline pH (9 & 11) due to the unavailability of electrons to participate in radiative recombination. The protonation of several carboxylic functional groups available at the surface of Cy@CD resulted in electron deficiency to exhibit substantial PL emission.

3.2.5 Cell viability/MTT assay

It is essential to assess the toxicity of NSCD to bacteria cells and hBECs by performing MTT assay to explore the promising application of NSCD in biological samples. This was carried out with NSCD tagged bacteria cells with concentration ranges from 0 µg mL^{-1} to 2200 µg mL^{-1} for 24 hours, as shown in Fig. 3.10. The viability percentage was calculated according to Equation 2.2.

The viability of bacterial cells in the absence and presence of NSCD has been closely monitored. After 24 hours of incubation of bacteria cells with and without NSCD showed a percentage viability of almost 97%. But the viability of S. aureus in the absence of NSCD is 96%. This is because the microbial cell viability depends upon the medium nutrient availability. As soon as nutrients get exhausted, microbial cells enter the dead phase of the growth curve. Hence, the number of dead cells increases than the number of live cells leading to the reduction in percentage viability.

Nevertheless, MTT assay demonstrated that NSCD are non-toxic to bacteria cells. The remarkable property of NSCD makes it a potential candidate for bio-imaging of live cells as well as other biomedical applications. The cytotoxicity of Cy@CD against bacterial cells was also investigated. In brief, 10^8 bacterial cells were incubated with different concentrations of Cy@CD such as 3.6, 18, 36, 90 & 180 µg mL^{-1} for 24 hours. The incubated sample of volume 100 µL was aliquot in the multiple wells, and 10 µL of MTT (5 mg mL^{-1}) was then added to each well of the multi-well plate. The sample mixture was incubated for 4 hours at 37 ˚C. A cautious approach was taken while aspirating the medium, followed by adding of 100 µL of solubilization solution to each well for dissolving the formazan crystals. After 15-30 minutes of shaking on a gyratory shaker, the optical density of each well was measured at 570 nm using a multi-well plate reader. The percentage viability was calculated according to Equation 2.2.

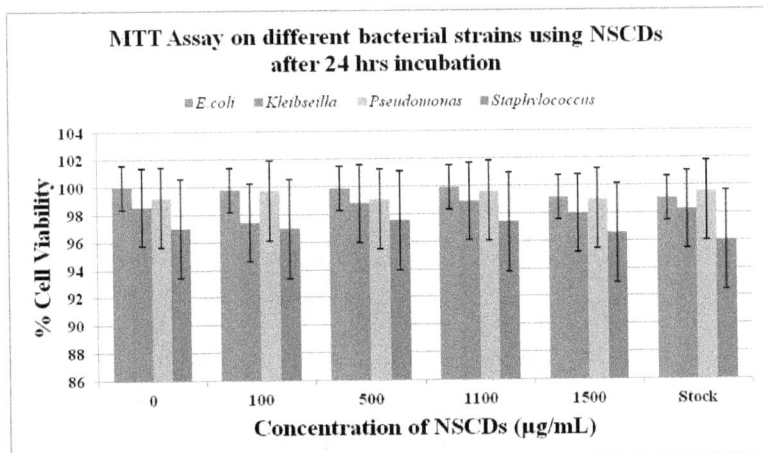

Fig. 3.10 MTT assay to check the cytotoxic effect on different bacteria strains by deploying various concentration of NSCD and incubating it for 24 hours

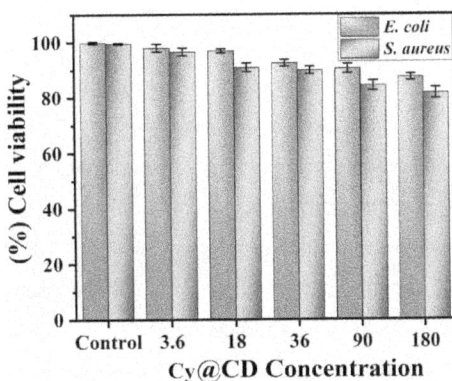

Fig. 3.11 MTT assay to check the viability of E. coli and S. aureus cells incubated with different concentrations of Cy@CD for 24 hours

The cell viability of *E. coli* and *S. aureus* were investigated in the presence of Cy@CD by using an MTT assay. Fig. 3.11 represents the percentage viability of *E. coli* and *S. aureus* cells after the incubation with different concentrations of Cy@CD for 24 hours. The outcome of the MTT assay exhibits more than 90% of cell viability even at the highest concentration of Cy@CD. This clearly demonstrate the biocompatible and non-toxicity of Cy@CD for microbial cells.

3.2.6 Cell imaging application of synthesized carbon dots in bacterial and mammalian cells

NSCD and Cy@CD were deployed to tag different types of cells as an application of bio-imaging. Several trials have been attempted to standardize the tagging protocol for various strains of bacteria and mammalian cells. We have discussed the imaging protocol in two different sections depending upon the cell type.

3.2.6.1 Imaging of bacterial cells using NSCD

Bacteria cells were tagged with NSCD and imaged under a fluorescence microscope at 40X magnification to probe the potential of bio-labeling properties of NSCD. Fig. 3.12A displays an excellent tagging efficiency with different bacteria strains used for the study. The figure includes a bright field image; the fluorescence image and overlay image consist of both bright field light and fluorescence light. Among all the available bacteria strains, *E. coli*, *P. aeruginosa* and *S. aureus* showed an outstanding tagging with NSCD. The bright field and fluorescence images were compared and established cell tagging. The cell internalization or endocytosis of NSCD happened when the cells were incubated with carbon dots and resulted in blue fluorescence when observed under a fluorescence microscope with a UV filter. Out of four bacterial strains, *K. pneumoniae* didn't show tagging with NSCD. The bright field and fluorescence images were compared and endowed the absence of tagged bacteria cells. The reason may be the catabolic characteristic of *K. pneumoniae* for different aromatic compounds and may result in decimation or disorientation of NSCD. Hence tagging efficiency for most of the bacteria strains were excellent, without trimming the fluorescence of NSCD. Such promising results clearly demonstrate that the NSCD synthesized in this work can be employed as a competent substitute for semiconductor quantum dots and organic dyes, which possess severe bio-toxicity issues and photo-bleaching.

66

The tagged *E. coli* cells were screened under different excitation wavelengths i.e., 380, 450, and 505 nm, and in bright fields by using NSCD as fluorescent imaging probes. The optical images were acquired at 430 nm (blue), 525 nm (green), and 590 nm (red) emissions. Fig. 3.12B illustrates a strong blue, green, and red fluorescence of *E. coli* cells observed after the incubation with NSCD for 3 hours.

3.2.6.2 Imaging of hBECs using NSCD

The competency of intracellular imaging of hBECs using NSCD as tagging agent was explored and showed in Fig. 3.12C. The NSCD tagged hBECs were observed under a fluorescence microscope at 40X magnification. The tagged hBECs displayed bright blue fluorescent under UV filter. Moreover, the nucleus of the epithelial cells was discretely tagged with NSCD. This can be explained as the cell internalization or endocytosis of NSCD helps it to migrate through the cell and cross the nuclear membrane to tag the nucleic acid component of the nucleus. As the size of the nucleus of hBECs is much larger than the size of a bacteria cell, the tagged nucleus was visible under the fluorescence microscope. Hence, NSCD can also be deployed for molecular studies such as DNA or RNA probing or protein estimation and perhaps a better substitute to the expensive commercialized biomarkers. The result suggests that NSCD has excellent biocompatibility and sublime cell permeability and can effectively apply to in vitro cell imaging and biological studies. These results implicated the potential ability of live-cell imaging of NSCD and can also be used to image various cells like cancer cells.

3.2.6.3 Imaging of bacterial cells using Cy@CD

The multicolour cell imaging of Cy@CD tagged bacterial cells (*E. coli*, *S. aureus*, *P. aeruginosa* and *B. subtilis*) and hBECs were carried out by using a fluorescence microscope. The tagged cells were imaged under different excitation filters such as 365, 450 and 525 nm. The bright field, fluorescence and overlay images of Cy@CD tagged *E. coli*, *S. aureus*, *P. aeruginosa* and *B. subtilis* cells were shown in Fig. 3.13A, B, C & D. The multicolour fluorescence from Cy@CD tagged bacterial cells were evident and can be explained on the basis of non-specific electrostatic interaction between the positively charged Cy@CD and negatively charged bacterial cells.

67

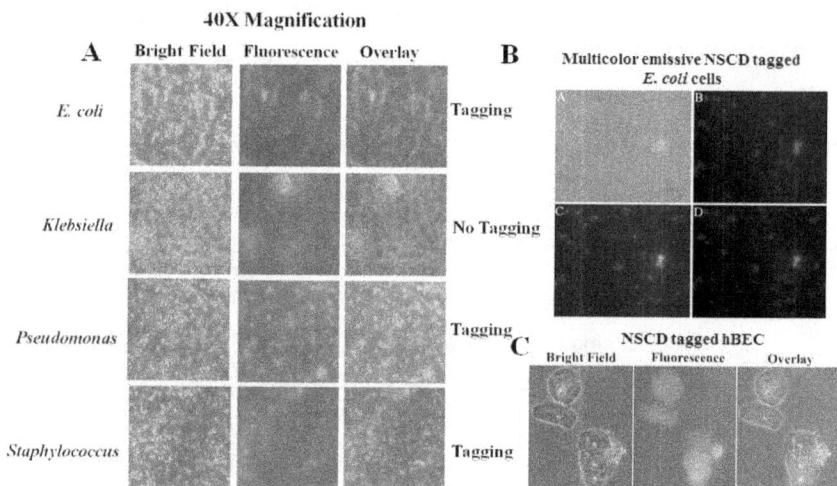

Fig. 3.12 A) Fluorescence microscopic images of tagged bacterial cells with NSCD (the image consists of bright field, fluorescence images, and overlay images of different bacterial strains), B) multicolour imaging of E. coli cells at the different excitation wavelength (380, 450 and 505 nm), and C) NSCD tagged hBEC at the bright field, fluorescent and overlay image (at 380 nm excitation)

3.2.6.4 Imaging of hBECs using Cy@CD

hBEC showed cell internalization of Cy@CD by crossing the cell membrane and tagging the nucleic acid of buccal epithelial cells (Fig. 3.14). The mechanism of cell internalization is based on macropinocytosis. Macropinocytosis is unique pinocytosis or cell drinking process having large membrane extensions. These extensions resulted in cytoskeleton rearrangement, due to which the formation of large vesicles takes place. These vesicles trap a large number of nanoparticles or carbon dots (Cy@CD). The intake or entrapment of Cy@CD is non-specific and would not be possible in the case of phagocytosis, clathrin, and caveolae dependent endocytosis pathways. The involvement of macropinocytosis pathways in passing the carbon dots through the cell membrane of adenoid carcinoma cells has been experim entally proven by Wei and co-workers [466]. The Cy@CD tagged hBEC were spotted by overlay merged images of bright field and fluorescence images (Fig. 3.14).

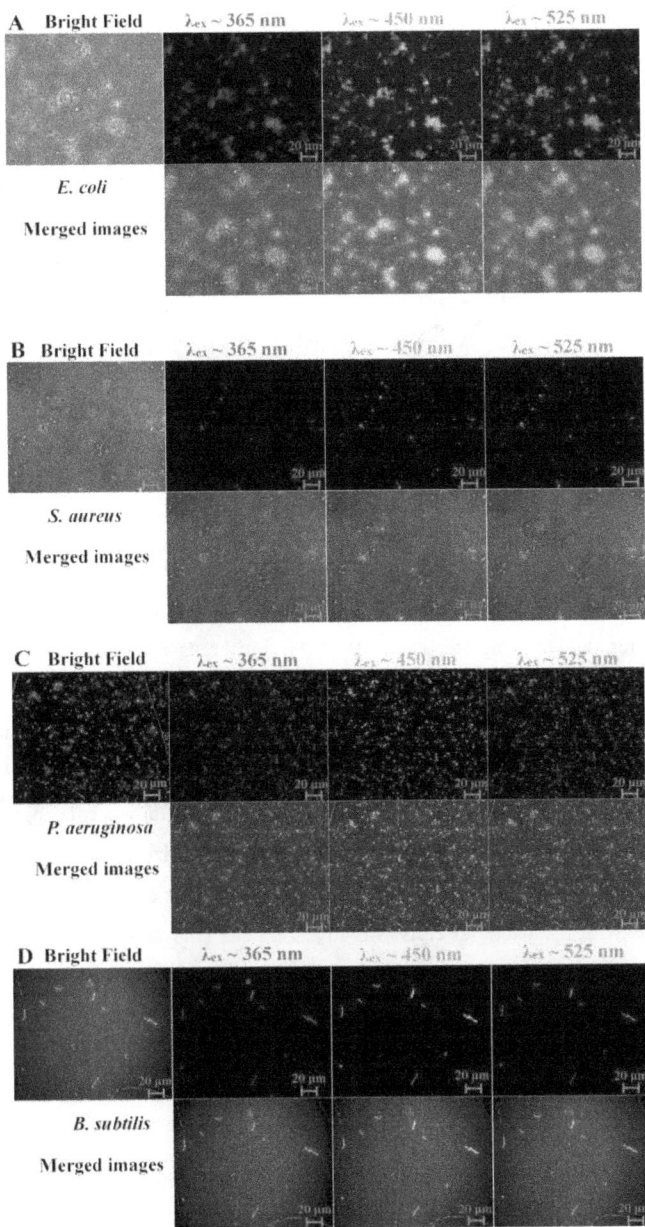

Fig. 3.13 Fluorescence microscopic images of multicolour emissive Cy@CD tagged bacterial cells viz; A) E. coli, B) S. aureus, C) P. aeruginosa, D) B. subtilis exhibiting blue, green, and red colour emission at different excitation wavelength (365, 450 and 525 nm) at 40X magnification

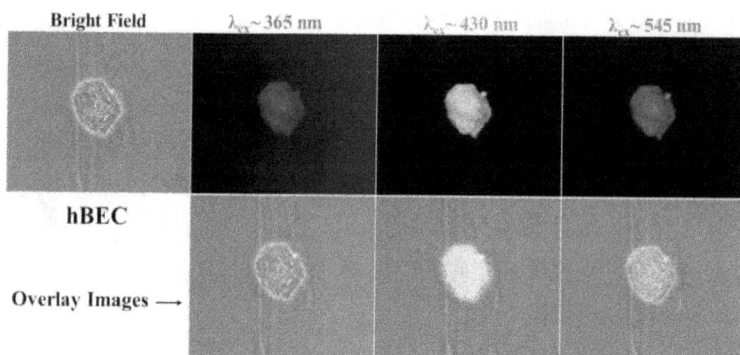

Fig. 3.14 Fluorescence microscopic images of multicolour emissive Cy@CD tagged hBEC exhibiting blue, green, and red colour emission at the different excitation wavelength (365, 450 and 525 nm) at 40X magnification.

3.3 Conclusion

A microwave-assisted hydrothermal method was used for the preparation of two variants of nitrogen and sulfur co-doped carbon dots from thiourea and 50X TAE buffer, and cysteamine and 50X TAE buffer as the precursors combination. The decent fluorescence quantum yields of NSCD & Cy@CD were estimated as 57% and 13.2%. The higher yield is due to the synergistic effect of nitrogen and sulfur dopants. The monodispersed N/S co-doped carbon dots were used for direct tagging of different bacterial strains and hBECs with superior fluorescence signals. The property of cell internalization or endocytosis of the synthesized carbon dots was observed in bacterial strains as well as hBECs. The multicolour emission property of the carbon dots with the bacterial cells was investigated. This was achieved by imaging tagged bacterial cells under different excitation filters such as UV, blue and green filters. Both the variants of N/ S co-doped carbon dots have shown effective tagging with varieties of cells and can become a suitable option for the expensive and harmful commercial fluorophores.

Chapter 4

***Facile pH-sensitive optical detection of
pathogenic bacteria and cell imaging using
multi-emissive nitrogen-doped carbon dots***

4. Facile pH-sensitive optical detection of pathogenic bacteria and cell imaging using multi-emissive nitrogen-doped carbon dots

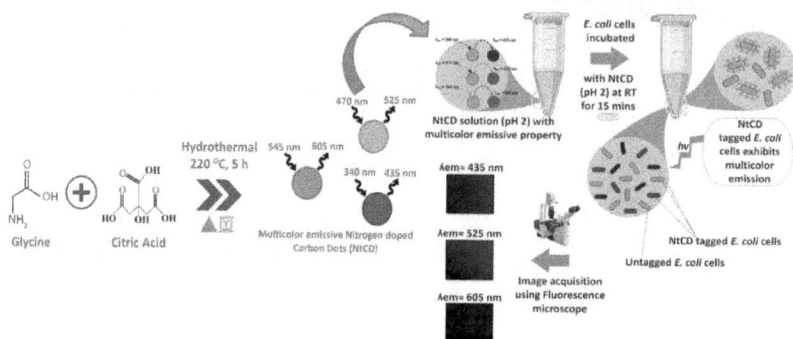

This chapter explains the facile one-step synthesis of pH-sensitive nitrogen-doped carbon dots (NtCD) to image different pathogenic bacteria and mammalian cells. The NtCD was synthesized using citric acid and glycine as precursors having carbon and nitrogen sources. The electronic characterization of NtCD was carried out by analyzing absorption and PL emission spectra. The NtCD exhibits significant PLQY (27.2%). The net charges present on the surface of NtCD, NtCD tagged *E. coli,* and NtCD tagged *S. aureus* were analyzed by a zeta potential (ζ) analyzer. The pH-sensitive pathogen detection using NtCD was explored by tagging different bacteria such as *E. coli*, *S. aureus,* and so forth at pH 2. Similarly, to explore the mammalian cell imaging potential of NtCD, SECs were employed as an ideal candidate. The NtCD tagged bacteria cells and SECs emit multicolour emissions after exposing it with different excitation wavelengths. The holistic approach of pH-sensitive tagging of NtCD with pathogenic bacteria provides a better insight into the efficient detection of lethal microbes in limited space settings. To the best of our knowledge, the pH-sensitive property of NtCD has never been attempted before to detect pathogenic bacteria.

4.1 Experimental methodology

4.1.1 Hydrothermal synthesis of NtCD

NtCD was prepared by using 2 g of citric acid and 0.62 g of glycine mixed thoroughly using mortar and pestle. This was finally dissolved in autoclaved Milli-Q water (5 mL). The solution was incubated in a hot air oven at 70 °C for 12 hours. The

71

thick syrup obtained after incubation was transferred into 100 mL Teflon-based autoclave for hydrothermal treatment at 230 °C for 6 hours. The heating rate was 15 °C min^{-1}. As the reaction completed, the temperature of the autoclave was slowly dropped to room temperature (RT). The resulting dark syrup after hydrothermal synthesis was diluted to 10 mL of Milli-Q water. The concentration of NtCD stock solution was 1.1 mg mL^{-1}. The stock solution of NtCD was centrifuged at high speed (at 14000 rpm) for 60 minutes to remove the unreacted impurities of NtCD solution in the form of a precipitate. The NtCD solution was further purified using a 0.22 micron syringe filter followed by dialysis (Molecular weight cut-off (MWCO) of the membrane = 1 kDa) for 48 hours in Milli-Q water. NtCD solution was diluted to a pale yellow colour solution (0.1 mg mL^{-1}) for performing cell imaging assay.

4.1.2 PL emission variation of NtCD & NtCD tagged bacterial cells at various pH

The fluorescence emission was scanned from 300 to 500 nm excitation wavelength to study the PL emission behaviour of NtCD. The disparity in PL emission of pH-sensitive NtCD was investigated at pH 1-11. The pH of NtCD stock solution was measured as 2. The precise changes in pH of NtCD solution were achieved by using standard solutions of strong acid (1 M HCl) and base (1 M NaOH). The PL emission peak of NtCD solution was gradually decreasing while moving down from pH 2 to pH 11. On a similar note, to study the PL emission response of pH-sensitive NtCD tagged bacterial cells, *E. coli* and *S. aureus* were deployed. The overnight grown bacterial culture was washed twice with PBS. The bacterial cell identification assay was performed by deploying NtCD solution (0.1 mg mL^{-1}) with pH ranging from pH 2-9. The washed cells were mixed gently with NtCD solution of different pH in a ratio of 10:1 and incubated at RT for 15 minutes. After incubation, the cells were washed with PBS so as to remove the unbound NtCD. The PL intensity of pH-sensitive NtCD tagged bacteria cells were measured at λ_{ex}= 340 nm, for which the λ_{em} was shifted from 435 to 415-417 nm wavelength range.

4.2 Results and discussion

4.2.1 Spectroscopic characterization of NtCD

The optical and electronic properties of water-soluble NtCD were examined at RT by using UV-Vis absorption and fluorescence spectrophotometer. The NtCD solution was transparent and pale yellow in daylight, but under UV light, a bright blue colour emission was observed (as shown in Fig. 4.1A). At different pH, the NtCD solution did not show variation in colour under daylight, but in a UV lamp, the PL intensity change was significantly evident (Fig. 4.2).

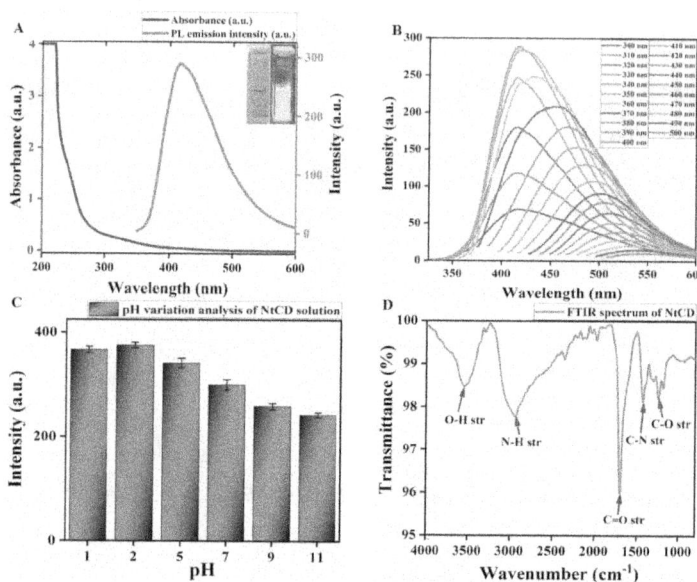

Fig. 4.1 (A) Absorption (blue colour plot) and PL emission plot (red colour) of NtCD. (Inset- Images of NtCD solution under day-light and UV light) (B) PL emission scans of NtCD at different excitation wavelength (300 to 500 nm) (C) Effect of change in pH (1 to 11) on PL emission response of NtCD (D) FTIR spectrum of NtCD

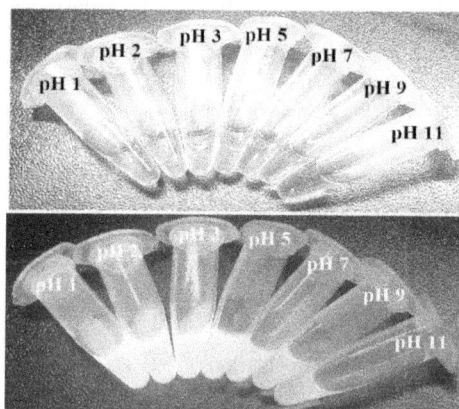

Fig. 4.2 Photographs of NtCD solutions with different pH under daylight (top) and UV light (bottom)

The NtCD solution was homogeneous without any precipitation at RT. The absorption plot of NtCD showed two shoulder peaks. The first peak at 260 nm is assigned to $\pi-\pi^*$ transition of sp^2 carbon domain. The second peak was at 340 nm wavelength is typically due to the n–π^* transition of the C=O bond. The fluorescence spectrum of NtCD showed maximum excitation (λ_{ex}) and its corresponding emission wavelength (λ_{em}) at 340 and 435 nm, respectively.

The calculated quantum yield (QY) of NtCD at pH 2 was as high as 27.2%. Similarly, the QY of NtCD was calculated at various pH (precisely from 2 to 11) to check the stability of NtCD (Table 4.1). The PL emissions scan at the different excitation wavelengths (300 to 500 nm) displayed a redshift while moving towards a longer wavelength (Fig. 4.1B). Hence, NtCD displayed excitation-dependent PL emission as one of its intrinsic properties. The theoretical concepts behind the aforementioned property can be the quantum confinement effect [342], surface traps model [467], or the electronegativity of heteroatoms[368, 468,469]. Perhaps, the prime reason is the presence of different emissive sites with an abundance of functional groups such as -C=O, -N-H, and -O-H on the surface of the NtCD, causing redshift [359].

Table 4.1 Percentage quantum yield of NtCD solution from pH 1- 11

pH of NtCD	Quantum Yield (%)
1	26.42
2	27.20
3	25.77
5	24.63
7	23.09
9	19.94
11	16.69

PL emission behaviour of NtCD solution was screened at various protonic conditions (from pH 1 to 11) as exhibited in Fig. 4.1C. The excitation wavelength was fixed at 340 nm. A significant variation in PL intensity was observed at discrete pH solutions of NtCD. PL intensity was highest at pH 2 (acidic environment) and lowest at pH 11 (alkaline environment). Apparently, the PL emission intensity at pH 1 and 2 were nearly identical. The reason could be proton saturation of the nitrogen sites in NtCD at pH 2 with no obvious possibility of extra proton attachment to the protonated NtCD nitrogen. Therefore, to achieve NtCD based bio-imaging applications, all the experiments were carried out at pH 2 (pH of stock solution). The variation in PL emission response can be described on the basis of pyridinic and pyrrolic nitrogen present on the surface of NtCD. The pyridinic nitrogen consists of lone pair of electrons on the outer side of the pyridinic ring and exhibits significant non-radiative recombination to quench the fluorescence by photo-induced electron transfer (PET) process [470]. Therefore, at low pH, lone pair of electrons engages in the formation of protonation complexes resulting in blocking of PET pathway and thus facilitates the fluorescence enhancement through local emission states [471,472]. The stated reason has been validated by an excellent response of PL emission to changing pH values (Fig. 4.1C). On the contrary, the radiative recombination process is evident in pyrrolic nitrogen due to the lone pair of electrons involved in maintaining the conjugation of the ring structure [471]. A significant upsurge in the fluorescence intensity was observed at pH 2. The gradual decrease in fluorescence intensity from pH 2 to 11 is due to the de-protonation of NtCD.

The de-protonation allows the pyridinic nitrogen to regain the lone pair of electrons and activates the PET pathway leading to quenching the fluorescence intensity of NtCD [472]. Furthermore, the protonation/de-protonation of NtCD at different pH was cross-validated by the zeta potential measurements. Thus, pH 2 was used as the 'tagging-pH' of NtCD solution to carry out the pH-sensitive detection of pathogenic bacteria.

4.2.2 Morphology characterization of NtCD

The morphological characterization of NtCD was carried out by using HR-TEM (as shown in Fig. 4.3A). The micrograph obtained showed many uniform, mono-dispersed, and well separated spherical carbon dots of size less than 5 nm. The TEM data revealed the fringe pattern (d-spacing of 0.21 nm (inset)), corresponding to the (100) lattice plane of graphite [473]. The size of the sixty spherical carbon dots was measured, and the size ranges from 1.20 to 4.62 nm with an average hydrodynamic diameter of 3.11 ± 0.75 nm as shown in Fig. 4.3B. Perhaps the variation in NtCD size explains the reason of the characteristic multicolour emission phenomena of NtCD.

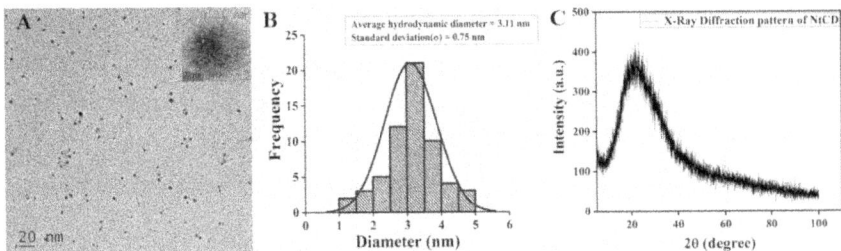

Fig. 4.3 (A) HR-TEM images for morphological analysis of NtCD (Inset: shows typical fringe patterns for d-spacing measurement of NtCD and was measured as 0.21 nm, Scale bar - 2 nm). (B) Histogram exhibiting the average hydrodynamic diameter. The size of NtCD was measured as 3.11 ± 0.75 nm. (Scale bar- 20 nm) (C) XRD pattern shows the graphitic carbon nature of amorphous NtCD

The XRD pattern of the NtCD, as shown in Fig. 4.3C, exhibits a prominent diffraction peak at $2\theta = 25°$. This was assigned to the highly disordered carbon atoms and further confirms the presence of graphite like carbon atoms arranged in stacks of disordered planes. Moreover, the XRD pattern reveals the amorphous characteristics of turbostratic carbon phase [474].

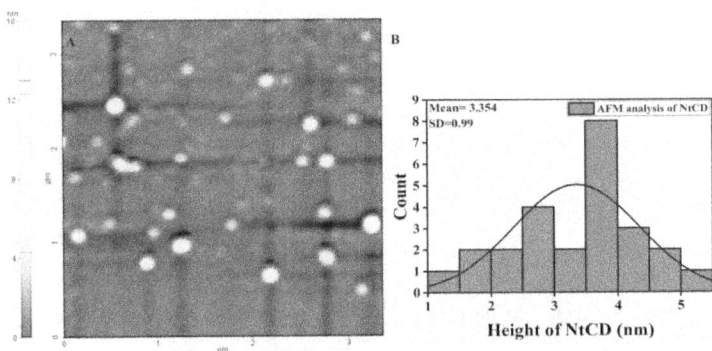

Fig. 4.4 A) AFM analysis of NtCD for the estimation of height profile and B) NtCD height distribution histogram

The height profile analysis of NtCD was achieved by atomic force microscopy (AFM) (Fig. 4.4A), and the calculated average height was 3.35 ± 0.99 nm (Fig. 4.4B). The significance of the NtCD height estimation (which varies from 1.3 to 5.5 nm) corresponds to the presence of several atomic layers of carbogenic graphene. The

AFM micrograph exhibited the uniform spherical morphology of NtCD. Such carbon atomic layer represent a graphite structure and has also been confirmed by XRD analysis.

DLS analysis was carried out to validate the hydrodynamic diameter of NtCD at different pH (Fig. 4.5). The NtCD size variation was measured as 1.03, 3.01, 17, and 71.2 nm at pH 2, 7, 9, and 11. This concludes that the bright NtCD emission at lower pH was from monomeric particles. The particles tended forming aggregates only at pH 9 and above.

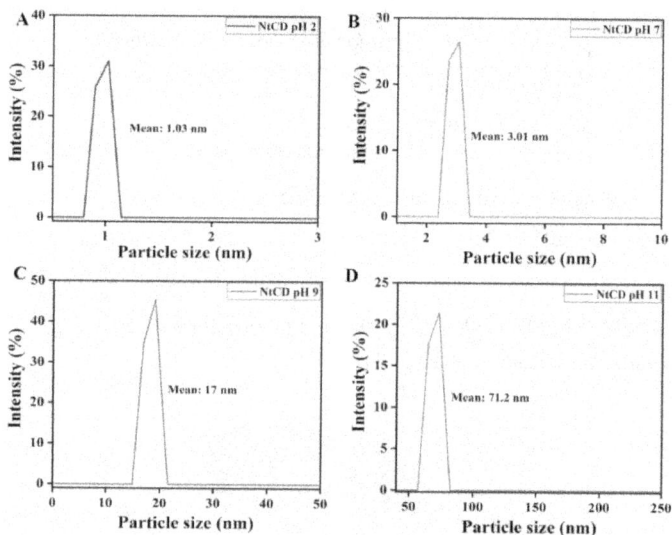

Fig. 4.5 DLS analysis for measuring the hydrodynamic diameter of the NtCD at A) pH 2, B) pH 7, C) pH 9, and D) pH 11

4.2.3 Chemical composition analysis of NtCD

FTIR spectrum of NtCD is shown in Fig. 4.1D and is typically used for analyzing the functional group available on the surface of synthesized NtCD. The FTIR spectrum of NtCD exhibits a broad peak at 3543 cm^{-1} and is ascribed to stretching vibration of the O-H group. The small peak at 2990 cm^{-1} corresponds to stretching vibration of >N-H and is primarily available due to the nitrogen doping provided by glycine. The absorption peak typically at 1695 cm^{-1} ascribed the stretching vibration of -C=O group of amides. The corresponding low intense peak observed at 1430 cm^{-1} is assigned to the –C-N group. The peak at 1236 cm^{-1} allocated to stretching vibration of >C-O group. The availability of O-H and >C=O groups confirms the hydrophilicity of NtCD, due to which it is highly soluble in water. The chemical composition of NtCD was further studied by XPS, as shown in Fig. 4.6. The wide scan result revealed that NtCD is comprised of carbon (C 1s), oxygen (O 1s), and nitrogen (N 1s), as shown in Fig. 4.6A. The atomic percentage is 77.66% for C 1s (maximum), 18.82% for O 1s, and 3.51% for N 1s, respectively. The de-convoluted XPS spectrum for carbon, oxygen, and nitrogen was explored. XPS spectrum of C 1s was de-convoluted to five peaks having binding energies at 283 eV for sp2 carbon, 283.7 eV for -C-C, 284.2 eV for –C-H, 286.7 eV for -C-O, -C=C, -C=N and -C≡N, 287.5 eV for O-C=O as exhibited in Fig. 4.6B. The high-resolution spectrum of N 1s (Fig. 4.6C) was de-convoluted to two peaks at binding energy 398.6 and 400.2 eV and ascribed to pyridinic and pyrrolic N. The de-convoluted high resolution spectrum for O 1s (Fig. 4.6D) shows two peaks at 530.3 and 531.5 eV which was attributed to organic -O-C=O and -C-OH. The result of FTIR and XPS was found to be an incomplete agreement with each other. Hence, the presence of N dopant on the surface of NtCD was confirmed.

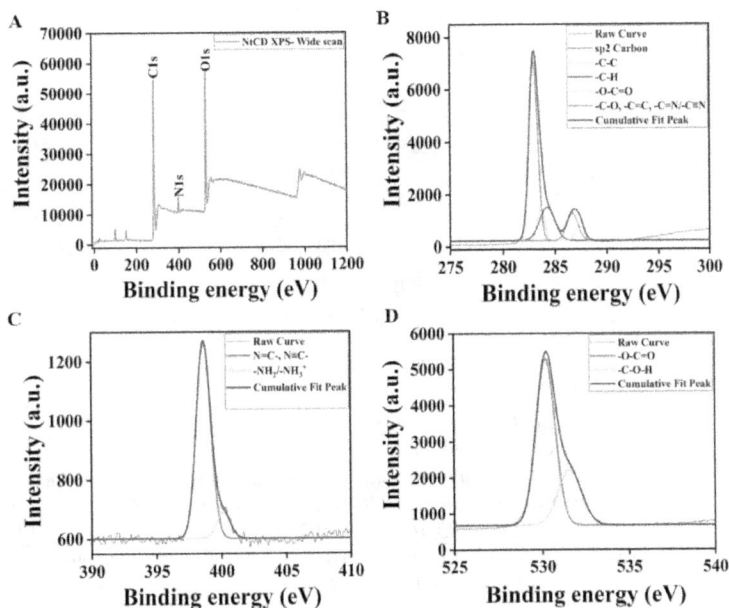

Fig. 4.6 XPS survey spectrum of NtCD, A) Wide scan of NtCD showing the elemental composition, De-convoluted spectra of B) C 1s, C) N 1s and D) O 1s.

4.2.4 Stability of NtCD at different conditions

The optical stability of NtCD was also investigated at different temperatures and ionic concentrations (Fig. 4.7A & B). The practical applications of NtCD can only be ensured on the stability of the novel carbon nanoprobes. The stability of NtCD PL emission was examined under several parameters such as temperature, ionic strength, time-dependent PL emission under continuous irradiation, and reversibility of pH changes. The PL emission stability of NtCD is examined for a wide range of temperatures (4−85 °C) and at a fixed temperature for 24 hours. The intensity of the NtCD was slightly quenched upon raising the temperature from 4 to 25 °C but relatively stable from 25 to 85 °C (as displayed in Fig. 4.7A).

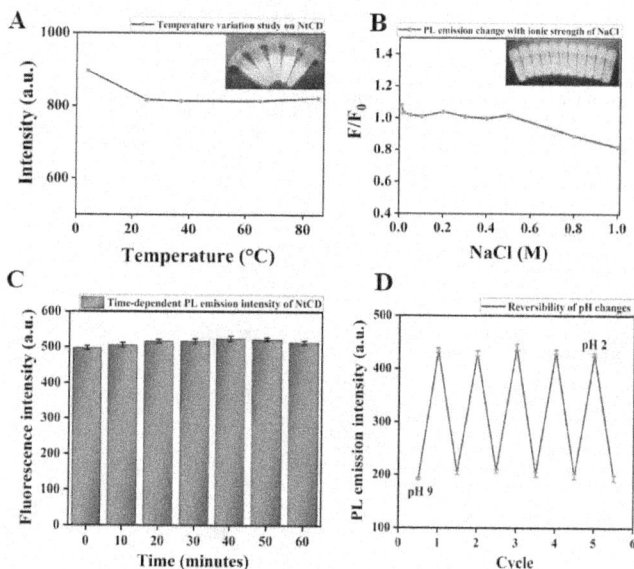

Fig 4.7 A) Effect of temperature variation on PL emission of NtCD (inset: PL emission of NtCD solution under UV lamp stored at different temperature ((4−85 °C)) B) Effect of various concentrations of NaCl on the fluorescence intensity of NtCD (inset: PL emission of NtCD solution along with different ionic strength of NaCl such as 0, 0.01, 0.02, 0.05, 0.1, 0.2, 0.3, 0.4, 0.5, 0.8, 1 M) C) Effect of time intervals of irradiation with a UV lamp on fluorescence intensity of NtCD. D) Reversibility of NtCD PL emission at pH 9 − 2 − 9 for five cycles.

The stability of NtCD PL emission was investigated from low to high concentration of NaCl (0, 0.01, 0.02, 0.05, 0.1, 0.2, 0.3, 0.4, 0.5, 0.8, 1 M). The NtCD solution was prepared under different ionic strengths of NaCl and was incubated at room temperature for 15 minutes. A feeble quenching of fluorescence intensity of NtCD was observed towards higher ionic concentration (0.5 M to 1 M), suggesting the stability of PL. The time-dependent fluorescence emission intensity of NtCD under continuous irradiation was also measured to screen the photo-stability of NtCD as shown in Fig. 4.7C. The time-dependent PL emission exhibits the stability of NtCD under continuous irradiation of UV lamp up to 60 minutes. The PL emission intensity was measured at an interval of 10 minutes, and observed the stability of NtCD without any significant variation in the fluorescence intensity.

In view of exploring the bio-imaging applications, the reversibility of pH changes in a biological system cannot be ignored [475,476]. Consequently, the reversibility of NtCD was investigated by monitoring the PL intensity change from pH 9 to pH 2 and again to pH 9 up to five cycles, as shown in Fig. 4.7D. It was observed that the variation in PL intensity was minimal and was quite stable even after five cycles representing the brilliant reversibility of NtCD.

4.2.5 Zeta potential study of NtCD

The zeta potential of NtCD (prepared in 0.1 M PBS) at pH 2, 5, 7, 9 and 11 was measured as -5.2, -8.4, -9.5, -11.9 and -14.9 mV (Fig. 4.8). The magnitude of the negative charge is not high and is near to neutral for NtCD. The zeta potential of E. coli and S. aureus was measured as -18.4 mV and -13.4 mV in 0.1 M PBS solution. The negative charge on E. coli (Gram-negative bacteria) is slightly higher than S. aureus (Gram-positive bacteria) due to the presence of thick lipopolysaccharides/ endotoxin and peptidoglycan layer. In the case of S. aureus the thin peptidoglycan layer is incorporated with an anionic moiety known as teichoic acid, and the net negative charge was lesser than E. coli [477]. At pH 2, the surface of NtCD consists of protonated amino groups resulting in the electrostatic interaction with the negatively charged E. coli and S. aureus. Despite the fact that both the bacterial species consist of negative charges, NtCD showed higher electrostatic interaction with E. coli than S. aureus. This can be attributed to the higher magnitude of negative charge available on E. coli cells. This results in the accumulation of excessive protonated NtCD in close proximity to the bacteria cells. The zeta potential of E. coli-NtCD mixture at pH 2 was -7.7 mV. This decrease in zeta potential establishes the existence of electrostatic interaction between protonated NtCD and E. coli. A similar explanation is applicable to protonated NtCD and *S. aureus* interaction. As pH changes from 2 to 9, de-protonation occurs, resulting in poor electrostatic interaction between NtCD tagged bacterial cells and is also evident in zeta potential analysis. The zeta potential results were in close agreement with the PL emission and fluorescence imaging results of the NtCD-bacteria mixture at different pH.

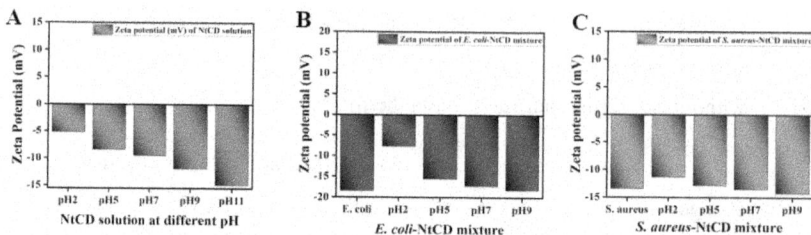

Fig. 4.8 Zeta potential analysis of A) NtCD (pH2 to 11), B) E. coli-NtCD mixture and C) S. aureus-NtCD mixture at pH 2 to 9

4.2.6 Mechanistic implications to study PL emission behaviour of NtCD tagged bacterial cells with pH change

The variation in PL emission response of NtCD tagged bacteria cells were analyzed at different pH. The highest PL emission of the tagged bacterial cells was observed at pH 2. The intensity of PL emission at pH 2 for NtCD tagged *E. coli* cells was greater than NtCD tagged *S. aureus* cells, respectively, and it follows a similar trend at different pH as well as shown in Fig. 4.9A. The reason could be the availability of NtCD in close proximity to the bacterial cells. The zeta potential of *E. coli* is more negative (-18.4 mV) as compared to *S. aureus* (-13.4 mV). Therefore, the protonated NtCD ($\zeta \sim$ -8.4 mV), at pH 2, shows higher electrostatic interaction with *E. coli* than *S. aureus* cells. The interaction results in lowering of net charge available on NtCD tagged *E. coli* mixture than NtCD tagged *S. aureus* mixture. This is because at pH 2, more number of protonated-NtCD molecules comes closer to *E. coli,* and the net charge reduces to $\zeta \sim$ -7.7 mV. The net negative charge is higher in the case of NtCD tagged *S. aureus* cells (-12.8 mV) which clearly indicates the weaker electrostatic interaction as shown in Fig. 4.9B. Hence, NtCD tagged *E. coli* cells were appeared to be distinct and brighter than NtCD tagged *S. aureus* cells. With the increase in pH from 2 to 7, the N-rich functional group present on the surface of NtCD gets de-protonated. This results in deprivation of electrostatic interaction between NtCD and bacteria. Furthermore, the tagging efficiency of NtCD with

81

bacteria cells was compromised with subdued PL emission response when the pH changed from 2 to 7. Perhaps the suggested mechanism provides the conceptual apprehension of PL emission behaviour of NtCD tagged *E. coli* and *S. aureus* cells at varying pH for detecting different types of microbes effectively.

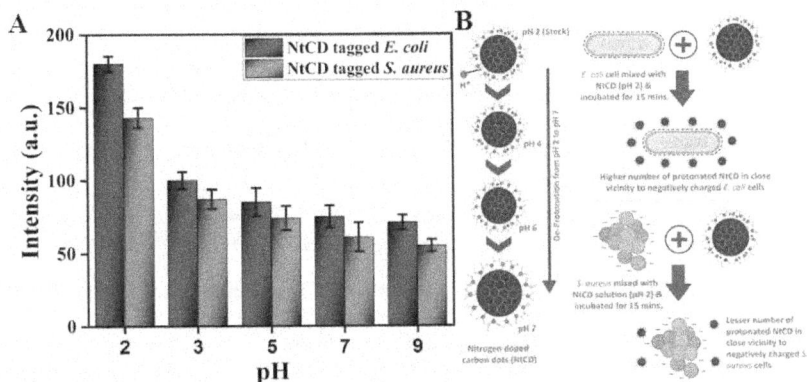

Fig. 4.9 (A) PL emission response of NtCD tagged bacteria cells at different pH and (B) schematic representation of the de-protonation mechanism of NtCD at pH 2 to pH 7 and characteristic NtCD tagging of E. coli and S. aureus at pH 2

4.2.7 MTT/ cell viability assay

The cell viability of *E. coli* and *S. aureus* were investigated in the presence of NtCD by using MTT assay. Fig. 4.10 represents the percentage viability of *E. coli* and *S. aureus* cells after the incubation with different concentrations of NtCD for 24 hours. The result of MTT assay explains the relationship between NtCD concentration and microbial cell viability. With the increase in NtCD concentration, cell viability decreases. It was observed that the highest concentration of NtCD leads to a steep decline in cell viability 57%) after incubating bacterial cells with NtCD for 24 hours. Perhaps the reason can be a well-known fact wherein a prolonged exposure of bacterial cells to an acidic environment results in cell lysing [478]. Here, at a higher concentration, the NtCD solution becomes acidic. At low pH, the acid tolerance of bacteria is significantly higher for the first 90 minutes, after which cell viability decreases gradually. Therefore, the histogram of MTT assay showed a dramatic reduction in cell viability of both *E. coli* and *S. aureus* incubated with NtCD for 24 hours.

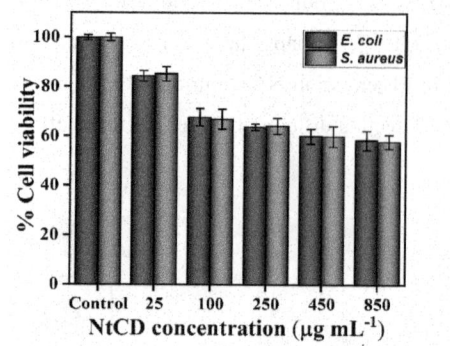

Fig. 4.10 Results obtained from the MTT assay on E. coli and S. aureus cells incubated with different concentrations of NtCD for 24 hours

4.2.8 Multicolour imaging of NtCD tagged bacterial and mammalian cells

4.2.8.1 Imaging of NtCD tagged bacterial cells

The competent multicolour imaging property of NtCD was tested by tagging it with several bacterial strains such as *S. aureus, E. coli, Bacillus subtilis,* and *P. vulgaris* at pH 2 (Fig. 4.11). After an incubation of 15 minutes with NtCD, all the bacterial strains were imaged using fluorescence microscopy. To cut down the possibility of auto-fluorescence, the untreated bacterial cells were used as a control, as displayed in Fig. 4.11A. NtCD treated bacterial cells with their overlay images have been shown in Fig. 4.11B. The tagged bacterial cells were imaged under different excitation filters such as 365, 470, and 530 nm with their respective blue (425 nm), green (525 nm), and red colour (605 nm) emission. Although the principle behind the multicolour emission has not been clearly demonstrated, there are two commonly proposed mechanisms. The first logical explanation is the usage of nitrogen as a dopant due to which surface defects are created on NtCD. It can be explained on the basis of functional group availability such as $-N-H$, $>C=O$, and $O-H$ on the surface of NtCD. This helps in creating additional energy levels in the form of emissive trap sites. The electronic transition varied significantly due to local emissive states with different bandgaps resulting in multicolour emission. The size variation of NtCD ranges from 1.5 nm to 4.8 nm (HR-TEM analysis) could be another feasible cause. The variation in size is directly related to an increase or decrease in the bandgap. As the bandgap increases, emission wavelength changes accordingly.

83

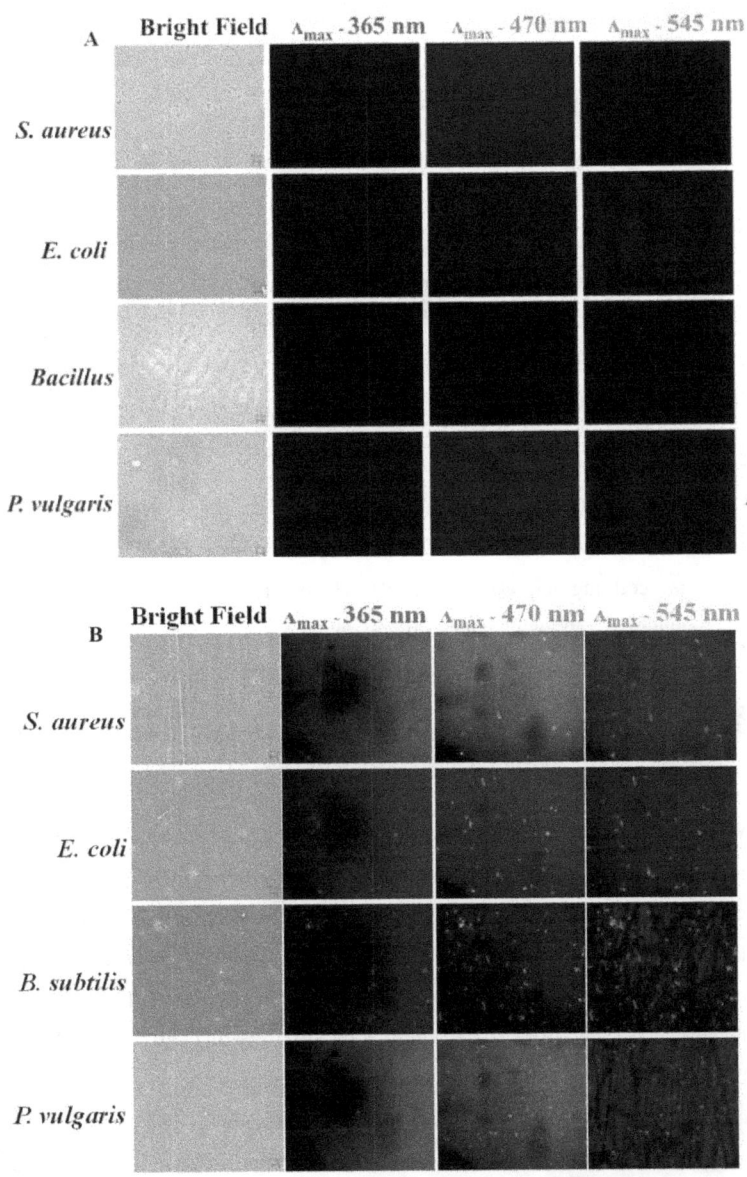

Fig. 4.11 Fluorescence microscopic images of A) untreated (control) and B) NtCD treated bacterial strains such as S. aureus, E. coli, Bacillus subtilis and Proteus vulgaris cells at pH 2 exhibiting multicolour emission (blue, green and red emission) with overlay images to spot the tagged bacterial cells

Therefore, multicolour emission was observed at varying excitation wavelength [479,480]. Hence, NtCD could be an ideal candidate for real-time and long-term imaging applications.

Despite NtCD showcased the cell tagging and imaging potential of an entire range of pathogenic bacteria, it experienced a few limitations which should not be ignored. The illumination, particularly at UV excitation, exhibits interference from biological/ clinical samples such as blood and urine, wastewater sample, and others. The biological samples have a strong background for both UV absorption and PL emission wavelength. A similar concept is realized for wastewater samples as well. The background fluorescence interferes with the illumination of UV excitation wavelength resulting in the weakening of PL emission signals.

Since NtCD possesses multicolour emission due to which the UV excitation can be switch over to blue and green excitation. This gives remarkable flexibility to bacterial cell tagging at specific pH. However, a stringent study is required to investigate the actions of interfering agents and to filter the background fluorescence to achieve the sensitive detection of lethal pathogens present in clinical samples.

4.2.8.2 Imaging of NtCD tagged Squamous Epithelial Cells (SEC)

The NtCD tagged SEC were imaged using a fluorescence microscope under various excitation filters as shown in Fig. 4.12. In this case, NtCD exhibits cell internalization or endocytosis due to higher cell permeability as compared to bacterial cells. The dimensions of SEC are 30-40 folds higher than a bacterial cell with the larger nucleus to cytoplasmic ratio. The NtCD was also permeable to the nuclear membrane, due to which it crosses the nuclear envelop and labels the available nucleic acid. The NtCD tagged nucleus of SEC was distinctly visible because of the bigger-sized nucleus. The NtCD capability of tagging the nucleus makes it a potent candidate for various investigations like nucleic acid (DNA/ RNA) quantification, protein estimation, and many more. The multicolour imaging of NtCD tagged SECs was attained once the labeled cells were illuminated with light of multiple wavelengths such as 365, 470, and 545 nm. The bright blue, green, and red colours were emitted from the tagged cells, and the images were acquired using a fluorescence microscope.

Thus, NtCD may provide an effective option for exorbitant fluorescent markers or dyes for probing mammalian cell lines such as cancer cells. With all these NtCD labeling capabilities, there is still a scope of investigation required for bio-imaging in clinical samples.

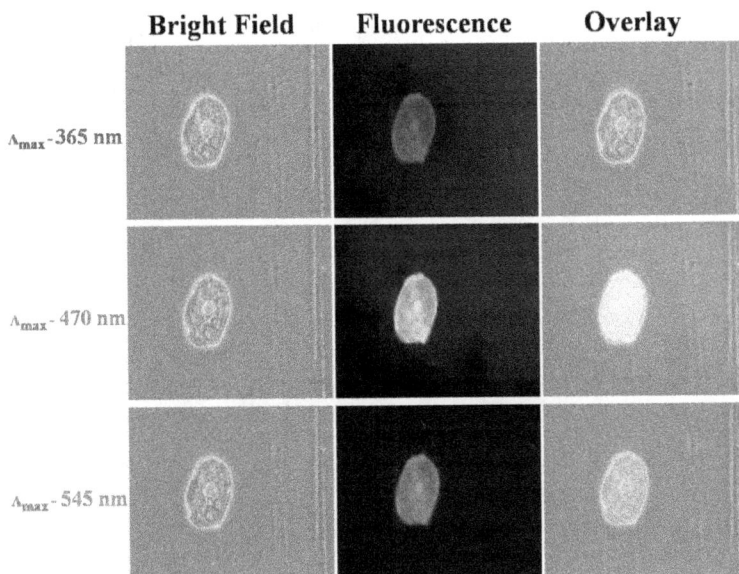

Fig. 4.12 Fluorescence microscopic image of multicolour emissive NtCD treated SEC at different excitation wavelength

4.3 Conclusion

In summary, a simple pH-sensitive detection method of pathogenic bacteria was developed using multicolour emissive nitrogen-doped carbon dots (NtCD). The PL emission stability of NtCD was probed at different temperature and ionic conditions to justify its robust nature. The PL emission was also tested at varying pH (1 to 11) and concluded the strong and stable PL intensity at pH 2 with high quantum yield (27.2%). The cell cytotoxicity nature of NtCD was tested by performed the viability test on two strains of bacteria. NtCD exhibited the relatable biocompatible nature of NtCD for cell tagging and imaging assays. The pathogenic bacteria such as *E. coli* and *S. aureus* were tagged with NtCD at various pH (2-9). It was found that the best 'tagging pH' was pH 2. The zeta potential analysis explains that the electrostatic interaction between NtCD and pathogenic bacteria facilitates the cell tagging assay. The unique multicolour emissive property was observed from NtCD tagged pathogenic bacteria and mammalian SEC for cell imaging. Therefore, NtCD could be utilized as an effective fluorescence probe in imaging bacterial and mammalian cells with brilliant photo-stability and excellent biocompatibility.

Chapter 5

Multicolour emissive colistin carbon dots based fluorimetric sensor for the detection of Gram-negative bacteria in real samples

5. Multicolour emissive colistin carbon dots based fluorimetric sensor for the detection of Gram-negative bacteria in real samples

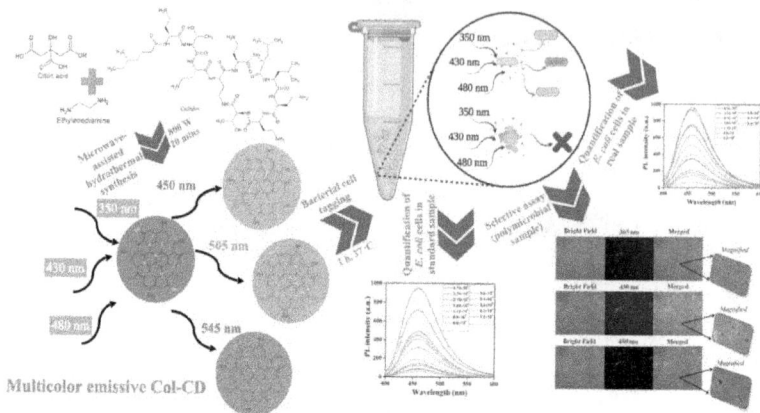

Multicolor emissive Col-CD

This chapter describes the selectivity of the synthesized colistin passivated carbon dots towards Gram-negative bacteria such as *Escherichia coli* and *Pseudomonas aeruginosa* as compared to Gram-positive bacteria like *Staphylococcus aureus* and *Bacillus anthracis,* and *Mycobacterium smegmatis.* Citric acid, ethylenediamine, and colistin were used for the one-step microwave-assisted synthesis of colistin passivated carbon dots (m-CCD) in a domestic microwave oven. Colistin is known to be a cyclic polypeptide antibiotic explicitly used against Gram-negative bacteria. The detection was performed by fluorescence microscopic and spectrophotometric analysis. The Gram-positive (*S. aureus*) and Gram-negative (*E. coli*) bacteria were used as model organisms for the specificity assay. The affinity of m-CCD was found to be higher for Gram-negative bacteria and showed a linear relationship in a wide range from 1.50×10^4 to 4.14×10^8 CFU mL^{-1} (R^2 = 0.980) with the detection limit 1.3×10^2 CFU mL^{-1}. The m-CCD was also used to screen Gram-negative bacterial cells in real samples such as tap water and urine samples. The detection range for tap water was analyzed from 1.50×10^4 to 4.90×10^8 CFU mL^{-1} (R^2 = 0.970) with the calculated LOD as 1.4×10^2 CFU mL^{-1}. The same analysis was carried out for urine samples with the detection range from 1.0×10^4 to 4.9×10^8 CFU mL^{-1} (R^2 = 0.931) with LOD 9.0×10^2 CFU mL^{-1}. Finally, the selectivity of m-CCD towards Gram-negative bacteria was confirmed by detecting *E. coli* cells in a polymicrobial solution.

5.1 Experimental methodology

5.1.1 Microwave synthesis of m-CCD

m-CCD synthesis was carried out using a mixture of 1 g of citric acid, 500 µg of ethylenediamine (EDA), and 15 mg colistin prepared in 5 mL autoclaved MilliQ water. The mixture was heated in a microwave oven for 15 minutes and then cooled to room temperature (RT). The charred mass was dissolved in 15 mL MilliQ water and then sonicated for 10 minutes. It was then centrifuged at 12000 rpm for 60 minutes to remove the un-reacted impurities. It was further purified using a 0.22 micron syringe filter followed by overnight dialysis using a 1 kDa dialysis membrane. The diluted m-CCD solution was pale yellow colour and was used for further assays.

5.1.2 Fluorescence spectrophotometric analysis of m-CCD tagged *E. coli* and *S. aureus* cells at different OD_{600} values

The selectivity of synthesized m-CCD towards Gram-negative bacteria was also screened at different OD_{600} values. The concentration of m-CCD was fixed (1:10 v/v) for tagging of *E. coli* and *S. aureus* cells. The m-CCD solution was mixed with the bacterial cell pellet and incubated for 1 hour at 37 °C. After the incubation, the bacterial cells were washed three times and finally prepared in MilliQ water to estimate the PL emission response. The fluorescence emission variation for m-CCD tagged *E. coli* and *S. aureus* cells at different OD was investigated at 350 nm excitation wavelength.

5.1.3 Selective recognition of m-CCD tagged *E. coli* cells in polymicrobial solution

The ability of m-CCD to identify the Gram-negative bacteria specifically in a mixture of two or more different microbial strains describes its remarkable selectivity. The polymicrobial sample was prepared by mixing *E. coli* and *S. aureus* cells. The target sample was prepared by mixing an equal volume ratio of both the bacterial cells. The pelleted cells of the polymicrobial sample were incubated with the m-CCD solution for 1 hour at 37 °C/180 rpm in a shaker incubator. Post incubation, the m-CCD tagged bacterial cells were washed twice to remove the unbound CD. Finally, the sample was prepared in MilliQ water and fixed on the microscopic glass slides with coverslips. The sample was analyzed at different excitation filters such as 365, 430, and 480 nm wavelengths; correspondingly, the fluorescence emission was obtained at 450, 505, and 545 nm, respectively. The microscopic images of selectively tagged *E. coli* cells over *S. aureus* have been acquired by using a fluorescence microscope at 40X magnification.

5.2 Results and discussion

5.2.1 Spectroscopic characterization of m-CCD

The spectroscopic properties of m-CCD were explored using UV-Vis absorption and PL emission spectrophotometer. UV-Vis absorption plot typically exhibits two ultraviolet peaks with a tail stretching to the visible region (Fig. 5.1A). The weak shoulder at 240 nm is assigned to $\pi-\pi^*$ of sp^2 carbonized domain. A relatively stronger peak at 350 nm corresponds to $n-\pi^*$ transition due to the bulk availability of nitrogen-containing functional groups and carbonyl groups having lone pair of electrons. The synthesized m-CCD solution was homogenous due to the presence of several polar functionalities such as hydroxyl (O-H), amine (N-H) and carboxylic (-COOH) groups, due to which the hydrophilic nature of CD improved drastically. The colour of the stock solution appeared to be dark orangish, but the diluted solution was pale yellow in daylight. The m-CCD exhibited stable, bright blue colour under UV light, as shown in the inset of Fig 5.1A.

The strongest PL emission peak (λ_{em}) of m-CCD was observed at 450 nm corresponding to the excitation wavelength (λ_{ex}) of 350 nm (Fig. 5.1A). The PL quantum yield (PLQY) was calculated to be 79%. The surface passivation of colistin moiety in the CD matrix resulted in enhanced fluorescence emission, which resulted in superior PLQY obtained. Furthermore, the PL emission scan was carried out at different excitation wavelengths starting from 300 nm to 500 nm, as shown in Fig. 5.1B. The excitation-dependent emission is the intrinsic property of the carbon dots and was noticed to be on the lower side in m-CCD. The PL emission scan at different excitation wavelengths exhibited a subdued redshift and was observed only at the longer excitation wavelength. While scanning from 300 nm to 410 nm excitation wavelength, the prominent redshift was missing and was noticed only while moving from 420 nm to 500 nm. This could be described based on the uniform particle size of the m-CCD. The variations in the bandgap were not available to induce the redshift at various excitation wavelengths. The second possibility is the availability of similar surface functional groups due to uniform surface oxidation and amidation of nitrogen dopant provided by EDA and colistin moiety. The passivation of carbon dots attained due to colistin moiety provides a bulk of nitrogen functionalized surface reactive groups. Therefore, tunable PL emission was present but not as significant as the traditional carbon dots exhibited.

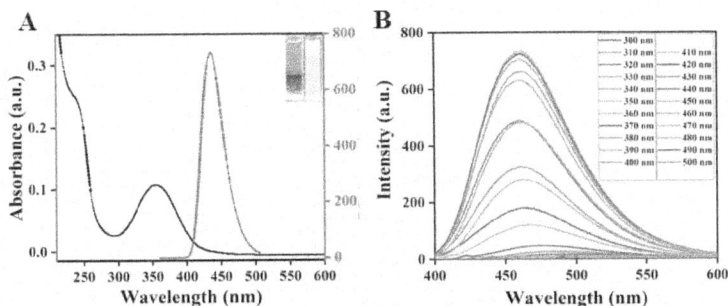

Fig. 5.1 A) UV- Vis absorption spectrum of m-CCD (black) and PL emission curve (red) ($\lambda_{ex}/\lambda_{em}$~ 350/450 nm) and B) PL emission scan from 300 nm to 500 nm excitation wavelength

5.2.2 Morphological characterization of m-CCD

HR-TEM micrograph of m-CCD exhibits mono-dispersed and uniformly spherical particles as shown in Fig. 5.2A. The average diameter of the synthesized particle was 4.6 ± 0.9 nm as judged from forty-five individual particles. The lattice plane of m-CCD is complementary to the plane of graphitic carbon (1 0 0) and is commonly assigned to turbostratic disorder in multiple stacked sheets. XRD analysis was also carried out to investigate the crystalline or amorphous nature of the synthesized m-CCD. The broad diffraction peak at 23.10° (Fig. 5.2B) corresponds to the amorphous characteristics of graphitic carbon as well.

Dynamic Light Scattering (DLS) was deployed to measure the average hydrodynamic diameter of m-CCD. The DLS measurements revealed the size of the m-CCD particles as 3.45 nm and revoked the possibility of aggregation of the synthesized carbon dots particles in the homogenous solution (as shown in Fig. 5.3). Thus, the DLS results were in close agreement with TEM results and validated the presence of mono-dispersed particles.

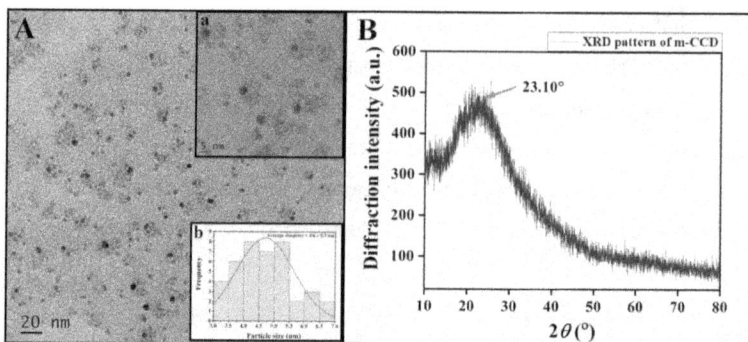

Fig. 5.2 A) HR-TEM micrograph of m-CCD exhibiting the uniform spherical particles (Inset a shows the magnified view of the spherical m-CCD) and the average diameter was measured as 4.6 ± 0.9 nm (Inset b displays the particle size histogram plot of m-CCD particles) and B) XRD pattern of m-CCD

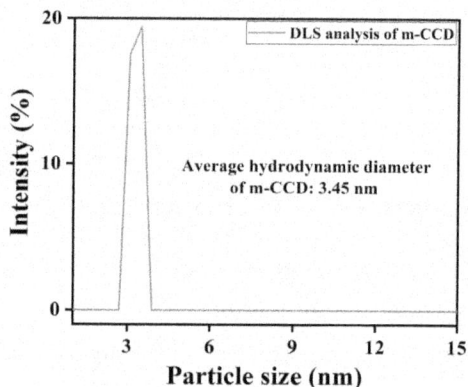

Fig. 5.3 Estimation of average hydrodynamic diameter of m-CCD using DLS method

5.2.3 Chemical composition analysis of m-CCD

FTIR spectroscopic analysis was carried out on the precursors and carbon dots variants such as colistin and m-CCD (Fig. 5.4) to confirm the surface passivation of colistin moiety. The IR absorption peak at 3180 cm^{-1} attributed to stretching vibrations of O-H and N-H functional groups due to the intramolecular hydrogen bonding exhibited by hydroxyl and amine functional groups. The small IR peak at 2900 cm^{-1} corresponds to stretching vibrations of C-H groups. The absorption peak at 1650 cm^{-1} corroborates stretching vibrations of the C=O functional group with a slight peak shift from the carbonyl functional group of colistin. This confirms the incorporation of colistin to the surface of synthesized m-CCD. The IR absorption peak at 1350 cm^{-1} attributed to the stretching vibrations of C-N in primary aromatic amine. The information revealed from the FTIR study needs to reaffirm with XPS analysis data to strongly validate the passivation of colistin residue over the surface of m-CCD.

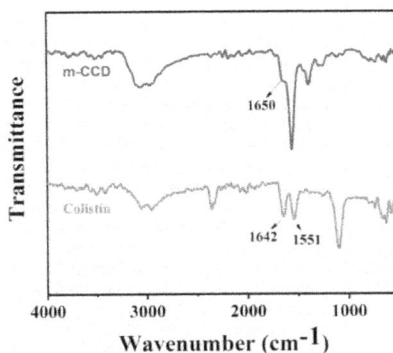

Fig. 5.4 FTIR spectra of colistin and m-CCD

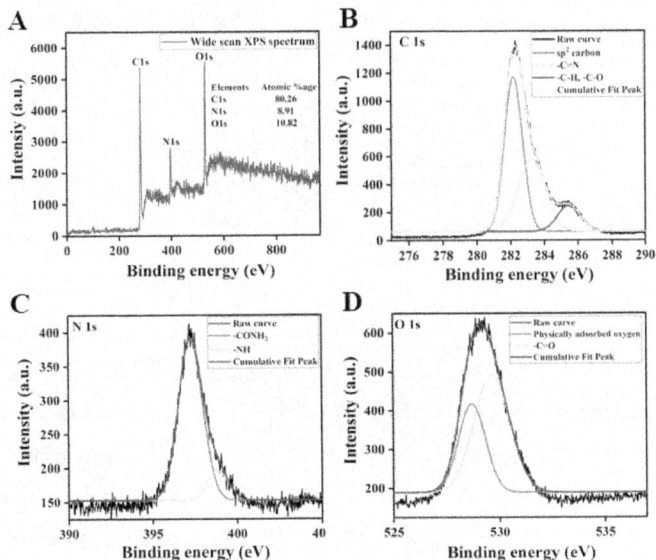

Fig. 5.5 XPS spectra of m-CCD showing the wide scan (A), high-resolution spectrum of C 1s (B) N 1s (C), and O 1s (D)

93

The wide scan XPS spectrum of m-CCD shows the presence of carbon (C 1s), nitrogen (N 1s) and oxygen (O 1s) at 284.5, 401.0, and 532.5 eV binding energies (Fig. 5.5A). The atomic percentage of C 1s, N 1s, and O 1s was measured as 80.26%, 8.91%, and 10.82%, suggesting sufficient nitrogen and oxygen elements for the intense fluorescence. The high-resolution scan of C 1s (Fig. 5.5B) exhibits the peaks at 283.18, 284.5, and 286.2 eV attributes to sp^2 carbon, -C=N and –C-H/ -C-O functional groups.

The de-convoluted XPS spectrum of N 1s (Fig. 5.5C) exhibited the peaks at 397.3 and 399.1 eV, which corroborates the presence of functional groups such –CONH$_2$ and amine (–NH). The high-resolution spectrum of O 1s (Fig. 5.5D) shows peaks at 529.6 and 530.7 eV and is assigned to physically adsorbed oxygen species and carboxylic (-C=O) functionalities.

5.2.4 Stability assay of m-CCD at different ionic concentrations, pH, and temperature

The stability of m-CCD was screened at different parameters to review the PL emission behaviour, as shown in Fig. 5.6A-C. The PL emission response of m-CCD was tested at different pH. The solution of varied pH from 2 to 11 was prepared by using standard 1 M HCl and 1 M NaOH solution. It was observed that the PL emission was highest at pH 7, with a subsequent reduction in PL intensity moving towards acidic or alkaline pH. Therefore, pH 7 was opted as the 'tagging pH' due to its highest PL intensity and also attained physiological condition for screening clinical samples.

The stability of PL emission was tested in the presence of different ionic strengths. NaCl solution was prepared with different concentrations starting from 0.1 M to 1 M. The fixed concentration of m-CCD was mixed with different concentrations of NaCl, and the variation in PL emission intensity was then investigated. There was no meaningful reduction or enhancement observed in PL emission intensities and hence stable at different ionic concentrations. The last stability assay was performed at a different temperature to check the PL emission variation. The storage temperature was 4, 25, 37, 55, 70, and 85 °C. Here also, the PL emission intensity of m-CCD was stable at different temperatures with no significant variations.

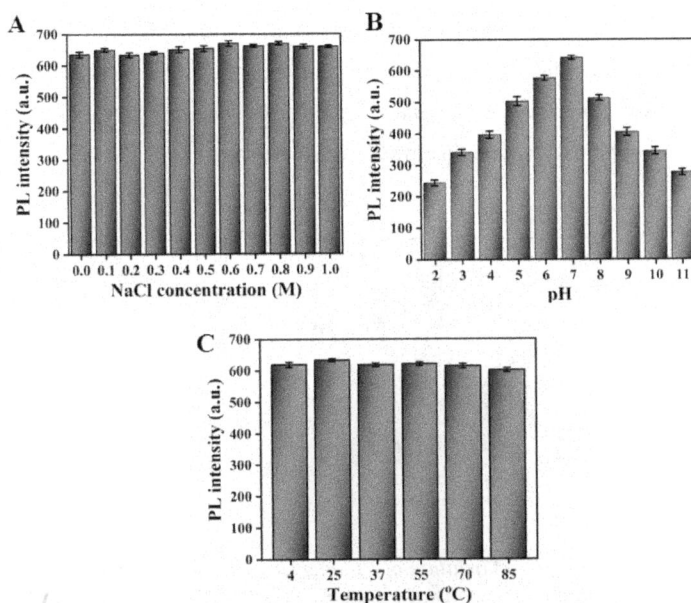

Fig. 5.6 Variation of PL emission behaviour of m-CCD with change in A) ionic concentrations (NaCl concentrations), B) pH, and C) temperature

5.2.5 Optimization of reaction time and colistin concentration for the synthesis of m-CCD

The m-CCD was synthesized using a domestic microwave oven at an optimized reaction time. The domestic microwave chamber was pre-heated for two cycles of 30 seconds each. The pyrolysis of CA/colistin/EDA in equal weight by volume ratio was achieved at different temperatures with a constant break of 20 seconds after every 5 minutes. This helps in controlling the chamber temperature and finally curbs the variations in the size of m-CCD post-synthesis. The reaction temperature was set at 5, 10, 15, 20, 25, and 30 minutes with constant time intervals. The brown-coloured charred mass was obtained after every reaction time other than 5 minutes. All the charred mass was diluted in fresh MilliQ water to dissolve the dried substance. Three rounds of sonication were carried out immediately, and the solution was centrifuged at 12100 rpm for 60 minutes to pellet down the solid impurities, and the supernatant was collected into the fresh vials. After centrifugation, the m-CCD solution was purified with a 0.22 μ syringe filter followed by membrane dialysis (MWCO: 1 kDa) for 24 hours. The PL emission of the purified m-CCD solution was screened by preparing 5 μL of CD in 3 mL MilliQ water. The PL emission of the m-CCD prepared at different reaction time is shown in Fig. 5.7A. The m-CCD prepared by 20 minutes heating exhibited the highest PL emission, and hence the optimum reaction time was fixed 20 minutes.

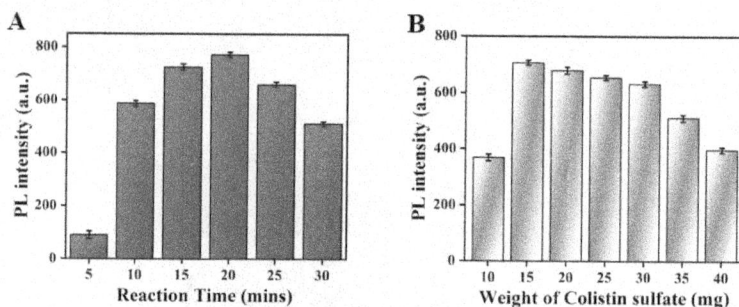

Fig. 5.7 Variation of PL intensity with (A) reaction time and B) weight of colistin sulfate required for the synthesis of m-CCD

The synthesis of m-CCD requires the optimum amount of colistin to achieve significant surface passivation. In addition, the surface passivated colistin moiety helps in enhancing the overall fluorescence emission. Therefore, the optimum amount of colistin was experimentally found out, as shown in Fig. 5.7B. Here, a different amount of colistin was added to the constant weight by volume ratio of citric acid (CA) and EDA. The weight of colistin varied from 10 to 40 mg. Post synthesis, the PL emission of different m-CCD was measured at 350 nm excitation wavelength. It was observed that the combination of 15 mg colistin with CA and EDA has a higher PL emission intensity as compared to the other weight proportion of colistin. Therefore, colistin with 15 mg weight was used in the synthesis of m-CCD with remarkable reproducibility.

5.2.6 Quantification of m-CCD tagged *E. coli* cells

The quantification of *E. coli* cells was achieved by investigating the PL emission intensity variation of m-CCD tagged bacteria at different concentrations in standard MilliQ water, as shown in Fig. 5.8. The PL emission response of m-CCD tagged *E. coli* cells was analyzed at 350 nm excitation wavelength. The broad detection range was calculated from 1.50×10^4 to 4.14×10^8 CFU mL^{-1} with a linear response ($R^2 = 0.980$) and a detection limit of 1.3×10^2 CFU mL^{-1} as shown in Fig. 5.8 (inset). The exceptional quantification demonstrates the tagging potential of m-CCD with Gram-negative bacteria specifically. The potential of m-CCD was also tested in real samples such as tap water and urine sample to screen the compatibility of the fluorescent probe.

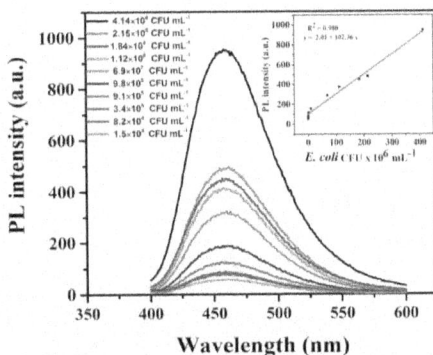

Fig. 5.8 PL emission spectra at different concentrations of m-CCD tagged E. coli cells present in a standard sample at 350 nm excitation wavelength (inset represents the linear regression plot of PL emission intensity with respect to E. coli concentrations)

5.2.7 Specificity of m-CCD towards *E. coli* over *S. aureus* cells

The PL emission signal of m-CCD tagged *E. coli* cells was higher than *S. aureus* and exhibited the selectivity of m-CCD towards *E. coli* (Fig. 5.9). The feeble PL emission intensity in m-CCD tagged *S. aureus* describes the poor interaction between the colistin moiety of m-CCD and the cell wall of *S. aureus* bacteria due to the absence of LPS membrane in Gram-positive bacteria. On the other hand, in the case of Gram-negative bacteria such as *E. coli*, the colistin moiety must have interacted with the LPS membrane present in the outer membrane of the cell wall. Finally, the interaction results in pore formation, due to which the permeability of the cell wall gets compromised, resulting in enhanced fluorescence emission. This corroborates the selective or specific nature of m-CCD towards Gram-negative bacteria such as *E. coli*.

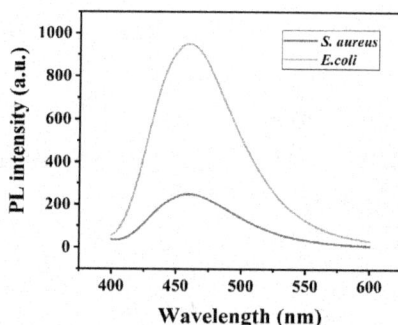

Fig. 5.9 PL emission spectrum of m-CCD tagged E. coli and S. aureus cells at 350 nm excitation wavelength

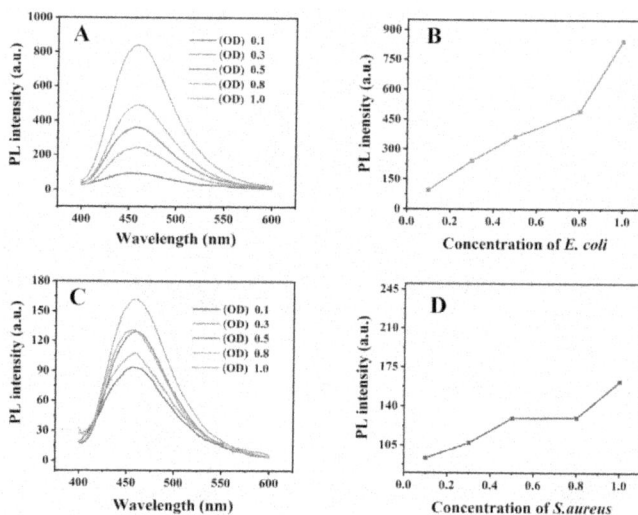

Fig. 5.10 A and C are PL emission responses of m-CCD tagged E. coli cells and S. aureus cells with varying OD_{600} values from 0.1 to 1.0 at 350 nm excitation wavelength. B and D are the concentration vs. PL intensity curves.

Fig. 5.10A and C exhibits the PL emission spectra of m-CCD tagged *E. coli* and *S. aureus* cells at OD values 0.1, 0.3, 0.5, 0.8, and 1.0, respectively. The variation in corresponding bacterial concentration-dependent PL emission intensities at 450 nm is shown in Fig. 5.10B and D. The outcome highlighted the enhanced fluorescence emission intensity of m-CCD tagged *E. coli* cells compared to *S. aureus* cells. The results suggest the selective affinity of m-CCD towards Gram-negative bacteria due to the availability of colistin moiety. Although the intensity variations are evident in both cases, the enhanced intensity in the case of Gram-negative bacteria demonstrates the selective nature of m-CCD.

Labeling studies were carried out using *E. coli, Pseudomonas, P. vulgaris, S. aureus, Bacillus* and *M. smegmatis* to justify the specificity of m-CCD towards Gram-negative bacterial cells in the presence of others. Fig. 5.11 exhibits the PL emission response of m-CCD tagged bacterial cells at 350 nm excitation wavelength. The PL emission was recorded highest for m-CCD tagged *E. coli,* and *Pseudomonas* cells. The m-CCD tagged *S. aureus, Bacillus* and *M. smegmatis* cells showed substantially low PL emission response. This explains the specific nature of m-CCD with a higher affinity towards Gram-negative bacteria. The lowest PL emission observed for Gram-negative *P. vulgaris* cells could be due to the natural resistance offered by the bacterial genome of *P. vulgaris* against polycationic colistin. The variations in emission intensity further highlighted the specificity of m-CCD towards Gram-negative bacteria.

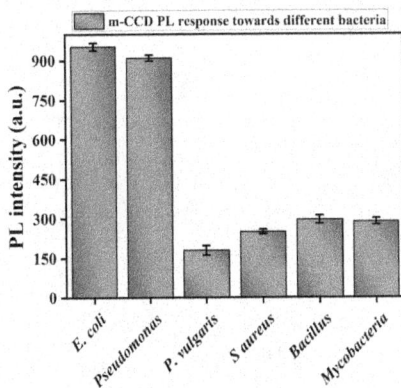

Fig. 5.11 PL emission response of m-CCD tagged Gram-negative and Gram-positive bacteria

5.2.8 Quantification of m-CCD tagged *E. coli* cells in real samples

The real samples such as tap water and human urine were collected in a sterile container and spiked immediately with the *E. coli* cells. The PL emission response of

99

m-CCD tagged *E. coli* cells in tap water was analyzed at 350 nm excitation wavelength using a fluorescence spectrophotometer. The fluorescence intensities of the tagged *E. coli* cells enhanced with an increase in bacterial cells. The broad quantification range of the m-CCD tagged *E. coli* cells present in tap water was calculated from 1.50×10^4 to 4.90×10^8 CFU mL^{-1} ($R^2 = 0.970$) with a detection limit of 1.4×10^2 CFU mL^{-1} (Fig. 5.12).

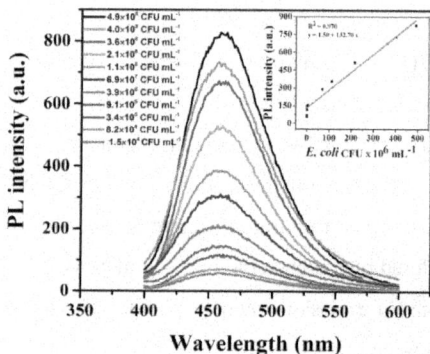

Fig. 5.12 PL emission spectra of different concentrations of m-CCD tagged E. coli cells present in tap water measured at 350 nm excitation wavelength (inset: the plot of PL emission intensity vs. E. coli concentrations)

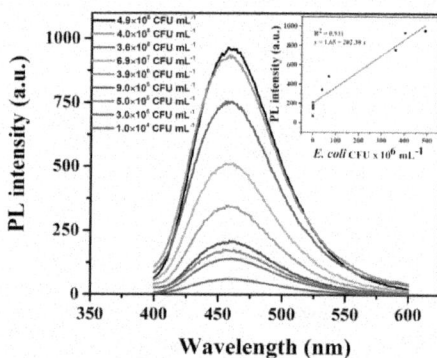

Fig. 5.13 PL emission spectra of different concentrations of m-CCD tagged E. coli cells present in human urine measured at 350 nm excitation wavelength (inset: the plot of PL emission intensity vs. E. coli concentrations)

The PL emission response of m-CCD tagged *E. coli* cells present in the human urine sample was analyzed at 350 nm excitation wavelength using a fluorescence spectrophotometer. The wide quantification range of the m-CCD tagged *E. coli* cells present in human urine was calculated from 1.0×10^4 to 4.9×10^8 CFU mL^{-1} ($R^2 = 0.931$) with LOD 9.0×10^2 CFU mL^{-1} (Fig. 5.13). These studies demonstrate the potential of m-CCD as a promising tool for detecting Gram-negative bacteria in samples of different matrices. The comparative analysis of the developed optical sensor in presence of standard and real samples (tap water and human urine) has been provided in Table 5.1

Table 5.1 Fluorimetric sensor performance in different types of samples

S. No.	Sample	Detection range (CFU mL^{-1})	Linearity	LOD (CFU mL^{-1})
1	Standard sample (culture)	1.50×10^4 to 4.14×10^8	0.980	1.3×10^2
2	Tap water	1.50×10^4 to 4.90×10^8	0.970	1.4×10^2
3	Human urine	1.0×10^4 to 4.9×10^8	0.931	9.0×10^2

5.2.9 Fluorescence microscopic studies

Fluorescence microscopic imaging was used to investigate the imaging potential of the m-CCD on various bacterial strains. Precisely, six bacterial strains, i.e., three strains of Gram-negative (*E. coli*, *P. aeruginosa* and *P. vulgaris*), two strains of Gram-positive (*S. aureus* and *B. subtilis*), and *M. smegmatis* bacteria were used to screen the imaging capability of m-CCD, as exhibited in Fig. 5.14.

The m-CCD tagged bacterial cells under UV excitation filter (~365 nm) exhibited intriguing results. The fluorescence imaging of m-CCD tagged Gram-negative bacteria such as *E. coli* and *P. aeruginosa* exhibited blue solid emission. On the contrary, *P. vulgaris* did not show blue emission because of the natural ability of the bacteria to resist colistin, having a specific genomic pattern to code for colistin-resistant proteins. The m-CCD tagged Gram-positive bacteria such as *S. aureus* and *B. subtilis* were also examined under UV excitation filter and were not visible. This proves the selectivity of m-CCD towards Gram-negative bacteria. In

101

the case of *B. subtilis* similar PL response was evident. The m-CCD tagged *M. smegmatis* bacteria also displayed subdued fluorescence intensity under the UV excitation filter. At different excitation wavelengths such as 430 and 480 nm, only tagged *E. coli* and *P. aeruginosa* cells were visible with bright green and red colour cells as shown in Fig. 5.14. On the other hand, m-CCD tagged Gram-positive bacteria, and *M. smegmatis* cells did not exhibit PL emission under both the excitation filters. This confirms the ability of m-CCD to image Gram-negative bacterial cells with multicolour emission selectively.

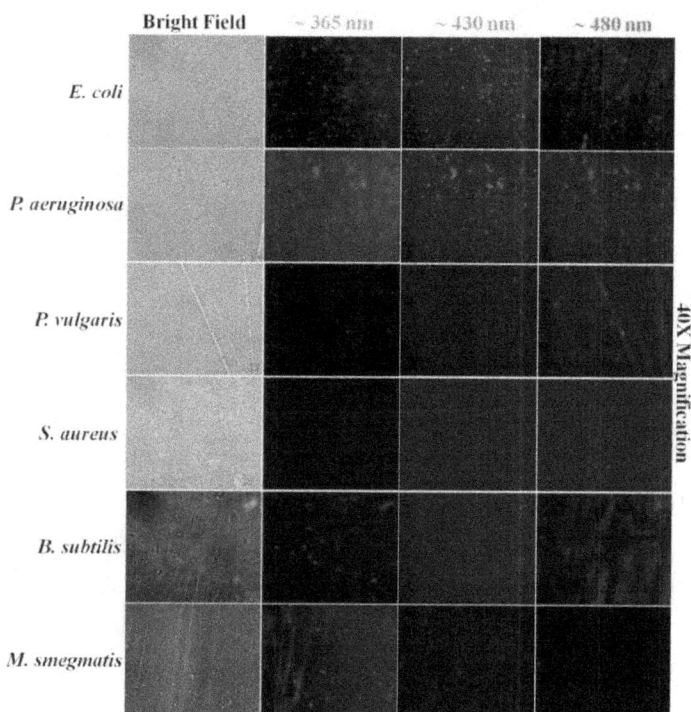

Fig. 5.14 Fluorescence microscopic images of m-CCD tagged E. coli, P. aeruginosa, P. vulgaris, S. aureus, B. subtilis, and M. smegmatis cells at different excitation wavelengths such as 365, 430, and 480 nm

5.2.10 Selective detection of Gram-negative bacteria in polymicrobial samples

The m-CCD tagged *E. coli* and *S. aureus* cells can be differentiated when observed under UV excitation filter (365 nm), as shown in Fig. 5.15. The m-CCD tagged *E. coli* and *S. aureus* bacterial cells under UV excitation were emitting blue colour but with significantly variable intensities. The m-CCD tagged *E. coli* cells were emitting with higher intensities as compared to *S. aureus* cells. Therefore, to prove the selective nature of m-CCD, the fluorescence emission of the tagged cells was explored with other excitation filters. The m-CCD tagged bacterial cells were observed under 430 and 480 nm excitation filters and displayed the prominent green and red fluorescence emission as shown in Fig. 5.15. This proves the selectivity of the synthesized m-CCDs towards Gram-negative bacteria such as *E. coli* in a polymicrobial sample.

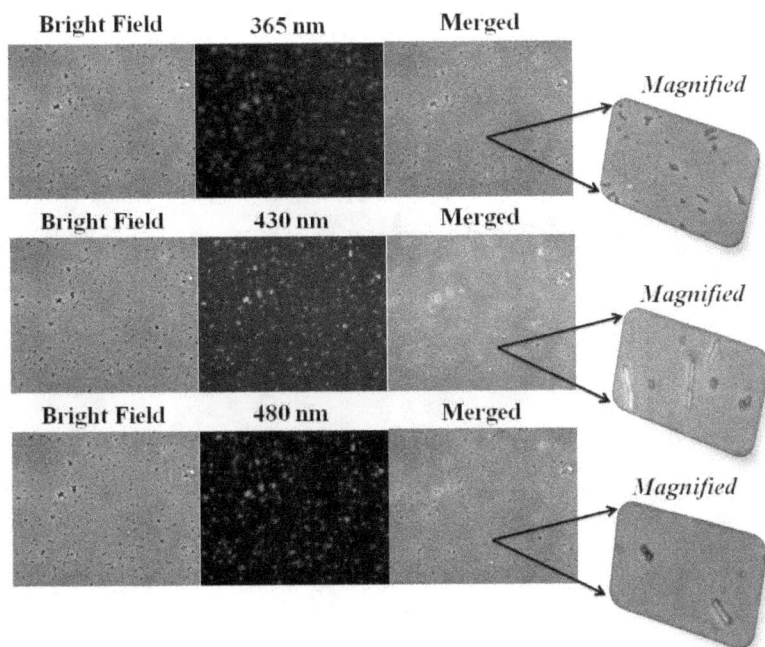

Fig. 5.15 Fluorescence microscopic images (under 365, 430, and 480 nm excitation filters at 40X magnification) of a polymicrobial solution consisting of E. coli and S. aureus cells incubated with m-CCD

5.2.11 Human buccal epithelial cells imaging using m-CCD

The tagging potential of m-CCD was investigated on mammalian hBEC. The human saliva sample was collected in a sterile container. The saliva consisting of salivary cells/hBEC was diluted multiple times using PBS to reduce the viscosity of the sample. The sample was centrifuged at a low speed (2000 rpm) for 8 minutes.

103

Finally, the salivary cell pellet was reconstituted in 400 µL of PBS. The hBEC and m-CCD were mixed in equal volume ratios and incubated for 15 minutes at RT. The intermittent mixing was carried out for achieving efficient tagging. The m-CCD-hBEC mixture was washed twice with PBS and then used for imaging. The tagged cell images were acquired using a fluorescence microscope under different excitation filters UV (330-380 nm), blue (450-490 nm), and green excitation (520-560 nm) at 40X magnification, as shown in Fig. 5.16. It was concluded that the m-CCD could also be used for mammalian cell imaging efficiently due to cell internalization and nucleic acid labeling.

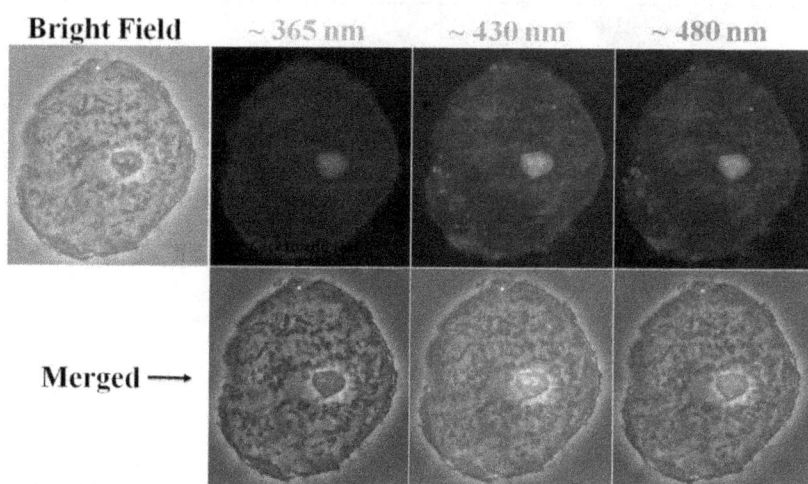

Fig. 5.16 Fluorescence microscopic images of m-CCD tagged hBEC viewed under different excitation filters at 40X magnification

5.3 Conclusion

In brief, the present work demonstrates the novel one-step microwave-assisted synthesis of colistin carbon dots as an efficient fluorescent probe for the specific detection of Gram-negative bacteria in standard and real samples. The PL stability assay of m-CCD was performed at different parameters such as ionic concentrations, temperature, and pH. The usage of m-CCD as an efficient fluorescent probe to be deployed as an optical sensor for bacterial detection was estimated by performing the quantification assay of Gram-negative bacteria. The m-CCD application for bacterial detection was also tested in real samples such as tap water and human urine samples, and the sensor exhibited a broad detection range and good linearity. The specificity of m-CCD was also screened in the polymicrobial sample and was highly specific to Gram-negative bacteria such as *E. coli* cells. Finally, m-CCD was also used for the imaging of mammalian cells such as hBEC. The m-CCD was tagging to hBEC and efficiently permeated inside the cell through endocytosis. The internalized m-CCD results in tagging the nucleic acid present in the cell nucleus. Therefore, the impeccable specificity, higher cell permeability and biocompatibility, and low cytotoxicity of m-CCD exhibit the potential to replace the conventional harmful organic dyes.

Chapter 6

Colistin carbon dots immobilized disposable impedimetric sensors for the ultrasensitive detection of E. coli in real samples

6. Colistin carbon dots immobilized disposable impedimetric sensors for the ultrasensitive detection of *E. coli* in real samples

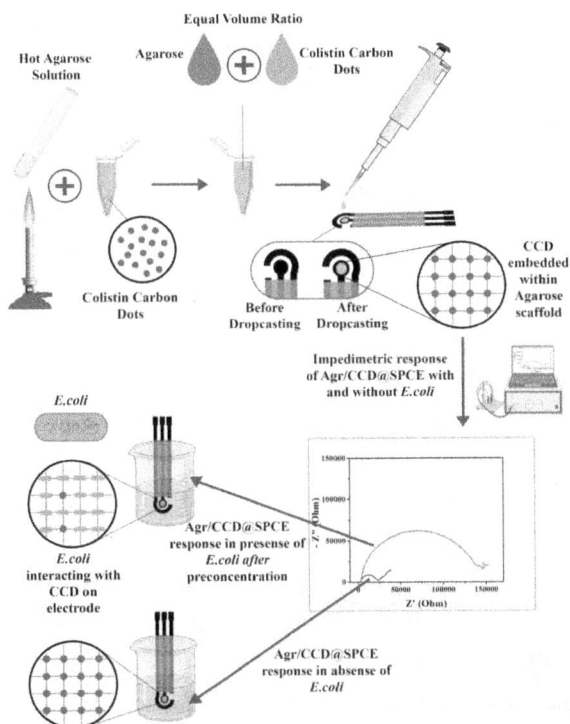

This chapter describes the performance of the novel, facile, label-free, and a cost-effective impedimetric sensor for the detection of *E. coli* using colistin carbon dots (CCD) immobilized agarose dried films on screen-printed carbon electrodes (Agr/CCD@SPCE). The interaction of *E.coli* with the modified electrode has been thoroughly studied using cyclic voltammetry, electrochemical impedance spectroscopy, and scanning electron microscopy. The quantification assay was carried out with a broad range of bacterial concentrations (10^2-10^8 CFU mL^{-1}) having linear regression, $R^2 = 0.98$, and the detection limit was calculated as low as 1.57 CFU mL^{-1}. The EIS response of Agr/CCD@SPCE was screened in a polymicrobial solution and was found to be highly selective for *E. coli* in the presence of other microbes such as *S. aureus, P. vulgaris,* and *M. smegmatis*. The selective nature of Agr/CCD@SPCE was due to colistin-modified carbon dots and has been cross-validated by the fluorescence microscopic studies using CCD-tagged bacterial cells. The sensor performance was also tested with real samples such as tap water and human urine with a sensitive response towards different concentrations of *E. coli*. The superior performance of the Agr/CCD@SPCE exhibits the potential of the sensor and exemplifies a promising candidate for the POCT of *E. coli*.

6.1 Experimental methodology

6.1.1 Hydrothermal synthesis of CCD

Colistin-based carbon dots were synthesized by using simple one-step pyrolysis of citric acid (50 mg), ethylenediamine (EDA, 20 µL), and colistin (10 mg mL^{-1}) at 180 °C for 1 hour. Here, citric acid acts as an efficient carbon source, and EDA provides nitrogen (N) atoms as a dopant to enhance fluorescence emissions. Colistin, also known as Polymixin E, is a polypeptide antibiotic and works efficiently against Gram-negative bacteria such as *E. coli*, *Psedumonas*, *Klebsiella*, and many more. The pyrolyzed CCD exhibited brown colour charred mass and was diluted in 10 mL MilliQ water. The CCD solution was centrifuged at 12100 rpm for 60 minutes to filter out the large particles present in the solution. This is the first step of purification. The supernatant was collected carefully and was further purified with a syringe filter (0.22 micron). The CCD was further purified by dialysis using a 1 kDa Molecular weight cut-off (MWCO) membrane to filter the ionic impurities. The colour of the purified solution was pale yellow, and it was used for the analysis.

6.1.2 Fabrication of screen-printed electrodes

Indigenously fabricated, screen-printed electrodes with three-electrode configurations as working electrode, carbon, and Ag/AgCl as counter and reference electrode respectively was used for the electrochemical analysis. The PET sheets were cleaned with acetone before screen printing and pre-heated at 90 °C for 30 minutes. A base layer of carbon ink and Ag/AgCl reference electrode was printed sequentially using an automated screen printer. The carbon ink was dried at 80 °C for 30 minutes, and the Ag/AgCl layer was dried at 80 °C for 15 minutes. The screen-printed carbon electrodes (SPCE) thus fabricated has the area of the working electrode as 3.14 mm^2 (r = 1 mm).

6.1.3 Preparation of Agr/CCD dried film and the fabrication of Agr/CCD@SPCE biosensor

The agarose solution (1%) was prepared in Milli Q water. Initially, different weight percentages of agarose were tested, and finally, 1% agarose solution was standardized for drop-casting over the surface of SPCE. The agarose solution was heated carefully to dissolve the agarose precipitate in water. The agarose solution was uniformly mixed with CCD in a 1:1 volume ratio by quick and vigorous vortexing. The homogenous solution (5 μL) of Agr/CCD was drop-casted over the clean working electrode surface. The Agr/CCD mixture was allowed to dry at room temperature for 4-5 hours. The dried film was firmly adhering to the surface of the electrodes and found to be stable enough even after dipping into the electrolyte solution. Various electrochemical and morphological characterizations confirmed the uniformity of the developed electrode (Agr/CCD@SPCE).

6.1.4 Microscopic characterization of Agr/CCD@SPCE

The microscopic validation of each modification step was performed using an Atomic Force Microscope (AFM, XE-70) and Scanning Electron Microscope (SEM, Carl Zeiss). The images of bare SPCE, Agarose drop-casted SPCE, and Agr/CCD@SPCE were acquired at different magnifications and scan size with better resolution. AFM images were acquired in non-contact mode within 6 μm x 6 μm scan area. Similarly, to acquire images at higher magnification and better resolution, SEM images were snapped at different magnifications. All the images were taken at 30.00 K magnification for each step of the modifications.

6.1.5 EIS experimental parameters

All the EIS experiments were carried out on electrochemical analyser (608D, CH instruments) using Agr/CCD modified SPCE. *E. coli* cells were pre-concentrated at the Agr/CCD@SPCE in 0.1 M PBS buffer (pH 7.4) at 0.5 V for 200 seconds. After pre-concentration, the CV and EIS measurements were performed using 5 mM $K_4[Fe(CN)_6]$ and 1.5 M KCl solution as a supporting electrolyte. All the experiments were carried out at room temperature. The impedance experiments were carried out in a frequency range from 1×10^5 to 0.01 Hz, with AC amplitude of 5 mV. The equivalent circuit and values of charge transfer resistance (R_{ct}) were deciphered by using simulation software (ZsimpWin 3.21).

6.1.6 *E. coli* detection and quantification using Agr/CCD@SPCE

The real-time monitoring and detection of *E. coli* were achieved by using Agr/CCD@SPCE for different concentrations ranging from 10^2 to 10^8 CFU mL^{-1}. All the experiments were carried out in triplicates to ensure the repeatability of the developed Agr/CCD@SPCE. New electrodes were used for all the concentrations, and R_{ct} values were obtained directly from corresponding Nyquist plots, and equivalent circuits were modeled using simulation software. The impedimetric detection assay duration was 20 mins and had a good fit to match the Point-of-Care (PoC) testing guidelines. The detection and quantification data obtained from Nyquist plots for different bacteria concentrations were statistically analyzed and represented accordingly.

6.1.7 Selectivity assay of Agr/CCD@SPCE in polymicrobial samples

Different bacterial strains were electrochemically tested, and the acquired values were analyzed to validate the selectivity of the Agr/CCD@SPCE. The bacterial strains used are *E. coli*, *S. aureus*, *P. vulgaris*, and *M. smegmatis* at the concentration of 10^8 CFU mL^{-1}. Individual Agr/CCD@SPCE was used to measure the impedimetric response for all the bacterial strains to cross-check the selectivity of the sensor in a polymicrobial solution. The R_{ct} values for the other bacterial strains were significantly different from the *E. coli* response. The polymicrobial solution was prepared with the known concentration of 10^5 CFU mL^{-1} bacteria viz; *S. aureus*, *P. vulgaris,* and *M. smegmatis* and varying concentrations of *E. coli*. The specificity of the modified electrodes was tested with the variations in the impedimetric response.

6.1.8 Real sample analysis

The application of the modified Agr/CCD@SPCE on real samples could justify its outreach to the end-user and also the commercial viability. The initial trials were performed using tap water and urine sample spiked with different concentrations of *E. coli* to screen the efficiency of the modified electrodes for the real samples. Fresh tap water and urine samples were procured and spiked with different concentrations of *E.coli* cells (10^3, 10^5, and 10^7 CFU mL^{-1}). There was no pre-processing required for both samples. The impedimetric responses for the different *E. coli* concentrations were measured along with the control (un-spiked). All the measurements were carried out in triplicates to justify the repeatability of the Agr/CCD@SPCE sensor.

6.2 Results and discussion

6.2.1 Spectroscopic characterization of CCD

The CCD synthesized by the hydrothermal method has been characterized thoroughly using various spectroscopic techniques such as UV-Vis absorption, photoluminescence (PL), IR, and XPS spectroscopy. The homogenous solution of CCD was transparent and pale yellow in daylight but bright blue under UV lamp, as shown in Fig. 6.1A (inset a).

The UV-Vis absorption spectrum exhibited two peaks (black curve in Fig. 6.1A). The feeble peak at 240 nm was attributed to the $\pi \rightarrow \pi^*$ transition due to the presence of sp^2 aromatic carbon. The intense second peak at 350 nm is assigned to n $\rightarrow \pi^*$ transition and indicates the bulk availability of lone pair of electrons on nitrogen and C=O functional groups at the surface of CCD [481]. The PL emission spectrum exhibits the highest emission peak (λ_{em}) at 456 nm corresponding to 350 nm excitation (λ_{ex}). The significant Stoke's shift between maximum excitation and emission peak was measured as 106 nm (Fig. 6.1A, inset b). The PL emission scan, as shown in Fig. 6.1B, was carried out from 300 to 500 nm excitation wavelength to obtain an insight into the luminescence behaviour of CCD. A redshift was observed while scanning from lower to higher excitation wavelength with a reduction in PL emission intensity.

A weak emission was noticed towards the longer end, due to which the intensity of multicolour emission was continuously decreased from blue to red. The subdued green and red emission could be due to the dominating blue emissive fluorophores known as (1, 2, 3, 5- tetrahydro-5-oxo-imidazo [1, 2-a] pyridine-7-carboxylic acid, IPCA [481].

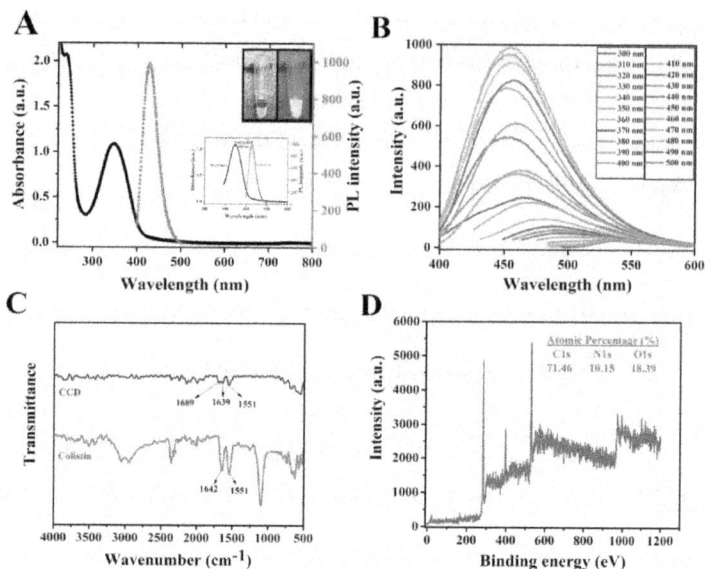

Fig.6.1 A) UV-Vis absorption spectrum of CCD with corresponding PL emission at 456 nm (inset a: photographs of CCD under ambient light (transparent) and under UV- 360 nm lamp (bright blue) inset b: A significant Stoke's shift between UV absorption peak at 350 nm and corresponding PL emission peak at 456 nm, B) PL emission spectra of CCD with different excitation wavelength, C) FTIR spectra of colistin precursor, and CCD and D) XPS wide scan spectrum of CCD

These fluorophores are formed due to condensation and dehydration reactions between citric acid and amine at low temperatures (140-150 °C) to form highly reactive amide bonds. As the temperature increases beyond 150 °C, carbon dots formation with carbogenic core takes place with high PL emission intensity [481].

6.2.2 Chemical composition analysis of CCD

FTIR and XPS investigated the chemical composition of CCD. The FTIR spectrum of the precursors and CCD were analyzed to confirm the presence of colistin moiety on the surface of synthesized carbon dots. The FTIR spectrum of CCD exhibits peaks at 1689, 1639 and 1551 cm^{-1} (Fig. 6.1C). The small peak at 1689 cm^{-1} corresponding to the stretching vibration showed by C=O functional group. This explains the amide bond formation on the surface of the carbon dot. The small peak at 1639 cm^{-1} attributed to the stretching vibrations of C=C. The peak at 1551 cm^{-1} corresponds to N-H bending vibrations. Therefore, the formation of an amide bond

111

confirms the passivation of colistin over the surface of CCD. The wide scan XPS analysis results exhibit three prominent peaks correspond to the presence of carbon, nitrogen, and oxygen at 284, 399, and 530 eV, respectively, on the surface of CCD (Fig. 6.1D)). The atomic percentage is 71.46% for C 1 s (maximum), 18.39% for O 1 s, and 10.15% for N 1 s, respectively. The de-convoluted XPS spectrum for carbon, nitrogen, and oxygen shows peaks at 285.11, 397.45, 398.82, and 530.01 eV and confirms the presence of -C-O, -C=O, -C=N, and -NH2 functional groups as shown in Fig. 6.2. The XPS spectrum of C 1s (Fig. 6.2A) was de-convoluted to three peaks with corresponding binding energies at 282.07 eV for sp^2 carbon and 283.21 eV for C-N 285.11 eV for C-H & C-O functional groups. The high-resolution spectrum of N 1s (Fig. 6.2B) was de-convoluted to three peaks at binding energy 396.66, 397.45, and 398.82 eV and ascribed to N-H, C=N and NH2 functional groups. The de-convoluted high-resolution spectrum for O 1s (Fig. 6.2C) shows two peaks at 528.51 and 530.01 eV which was attributed to physically adsorbed oxygen and organic C=O functional group. The result of FTIR and XPS was found to be in good agreement with each other. The XPS data revealed the surface functionalities of CCD and was found to be in close agreement with the FTIR data.

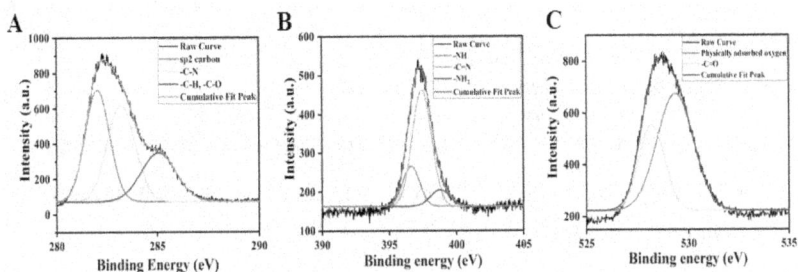

Fig. 6.2 The de-convoluted XPS spectrum of A) C 1s, B) N 1s, and C) O 1s to realize the presence of several functional groups on the surface of CCD

6.2.3 Morphological analysis of CCD

The morphological analysis of CCD was carried out by using HR-TEM. The micrograph displayed several near-spherical and mono-dispersed CCD with size ranges from 5-6 nm (Fig. 6.3A). The inset of Fig. 6.3A shows the definite fringe patterns with measured d-spacing as 0.20 nm, corresponding to the (1 0 0) lattice plane of graphite. The average diameter of forty CCD particles was calculated to be

5.41 ± 0.22 nm as shown in Fig. 6.3B. This attributed to highly disordered carbon atoms and confirms the availability of graphitic carbon atoms arranged in disordered planes.

The selected area electron diffraction (SAED) pattern (Fig. 6.3C) attained from TEM projects the diffused rings or halo devoid of any spots. This suggests the amorphous characteristic of the synthesized CCD.

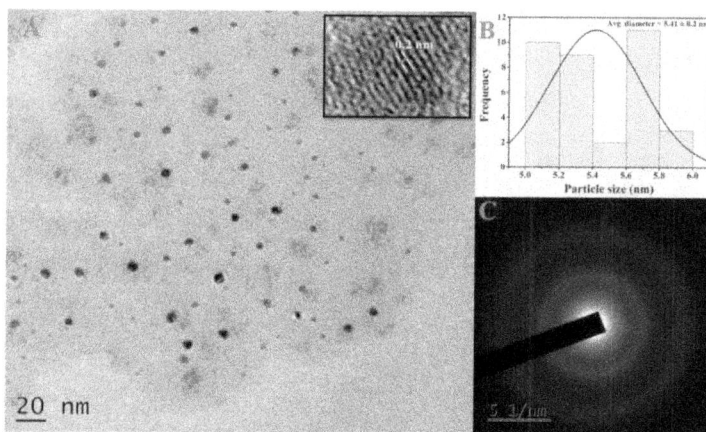

Fig.6.3 A) TEM micrograph of monodispersed spherical CCD particles (Inset: fringes pattern exhibiting measured interlayer distance of 0.2 nm), B) Histogram plot for measuring average size of forty CCD particles and C) SAED pattern of CCD showing diffuse rings corresponding to the amorphous nature

6.2.4 Fluorescence spectrophotometric analysis of CCD tagged *E. coli* and *S. aureus* cells

The fluorescence spectroscopy results of CCD-tagged *E. coli* and *S. aureus* cells are also analyzed and exhibited in Fig. 6.4. The specific nature of CCD was screened by labeling with Gram-positive (*S. aureus*) and Gram-negative bacteria (*E. coli*). The PL emission was observed at 458 nm, but the fluorescence intensity was highest for CCD-tagged *E. coli* cells than *S. aureus* cells. This justifies the specific nature of the synthesized fluorescent CCD towards *E. coli* because of the specific nature of polycationic colistin moiety of CCD towards Gram-negative cells.

113

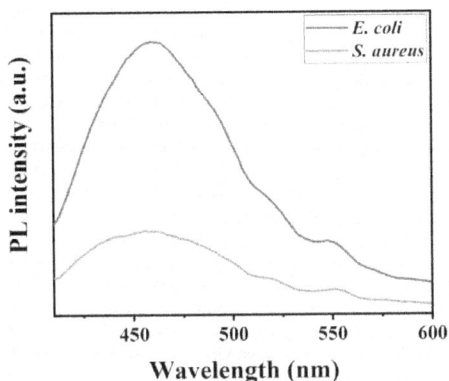

Fig. 6.4 PL emission spectrum of CCD tagged E. coli and S. aureus cells at 350 nm excitation wavelength

6.2.5 Fluorescence microscopic analysis of CCD tagged *E. coli* and *S. aureus* cells

The fluorescence microscopic investigation of CCD-tagged *E. coli* and *S. aureus* bacterial cells were carried out for achieving bio-imaging (Fig. 6.5A & B). The tagging was accomplished by mixing CCD solution with bacterial cells followed by incubation for 90 minutes at 37 °C. Post incubation, the solution was washed twice with MilliQ water, and the sample was fixed on a glass slide for image acquisition.

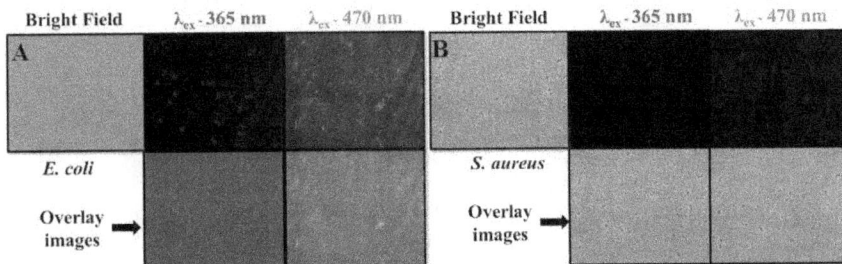

Fig. 6.5 Fluorescence microscopic images of CCD tagged A) E. coli and B) S. aureus cells at different excitation filters (λ_{ex} ~ 365 and 470 nm) with overlay images.

The CCD tagged *E. coli* and *S. aureus* cells were imaged separately under different excitation filters. The images show blue and green emission when excited at 365 and 470 nm, but there was no red emission observed at 545 nm excitation. This could be due to an insufficient degree of surface oxidation due to which bandgap variation might have resulted in blue and green emission only.

6.2.6 Characterization of Agr/CCD@SPCE

The spectroscopic, morphological, and electrochemical characterization of the modified electrode Agr/CCD@SPCE was achieved and discussed in the following sections.

6.2.6.1 FTIR analysis of Agr/CCD@SPCE

The involvement of various functional groups on each step of electrode fabrication was characterized using IR spectroscopy (Fig. 6.6). The blue curve represents the IR spectra of Agr@SPCE; it shows the presence of different functional groups such as O-H, C-H, and C-O. Apart from the different peaks observed in Agr@SPCE, the incorporation of colistin into the agarose film introduced a small peak of N-H bending vibrations at 1556 cm^{-1} and a dual peak at 3375, and 3259 cm^{-1} corresponds to N-H and O-H stretching vibrations. This shows the successful immobilization of CCD within dried agarose scaffold and its availability for sensing application. The daylight and UV lamp images of CCD immobilized/embedded within the agarose scaffold have been shown in Fig. 6.7.

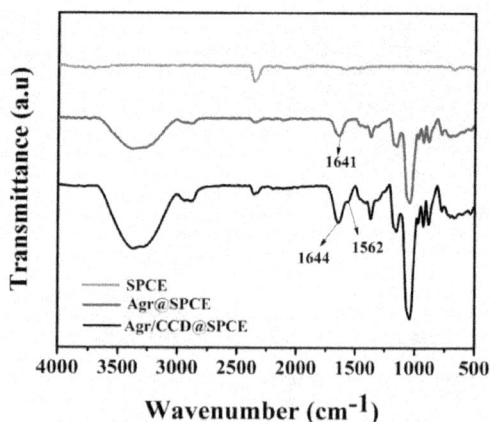

Fig. 6.6 FTIR characterization of Agr/CCD@SPCE to verify the presence of CCD within the agarose polymer scaffold by analyzing the presence of specific functional groups

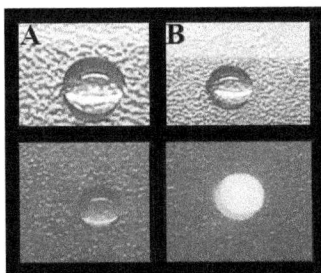

*Fig. 6.7 A) Bright light (top) and UV lamp (bottom) images of agarose only and B)
Transparent agarose intercalated CCD under bright light (top) and fluorescing under
UV lamp (bottom)*

6.2.6.2 Electrochemical characterization of Agr/CCD@SPCE

The systematic modification of the Agr/CCD@SPCE sensor was characterized by EIS and cyclic voltammetry (CV) to confirm the sensor construction (Fig. 6.8). The CV has been used to infer the redox behaviour as a function of input voltage, and EIS was deployed as a sensitive tool to study the charge transfer across the electrode-electrolyte interface.

The CV and EIS responses show the systematic modification of electrodes with and without the presence of bacteria. The overnight grown bacterial culture was washed twice and prepared in fresh 0.1 M PBS (pH 7.4). The bare and modified electrodes were pre-concentrated with a definite volume of bacterial samples. Since the bacterial cells are negatively charged, the pre-concentration parameters were defined accordingly. The applied voltage was set to +0.5 V for 200 seconds. The positive potential resulted in attracting negatively charged bacteria towards the surface of electrodes. Immediately after pre-concentration, the electrodes were subjected to CV and EIS in ferricyanide solution. The CV was carried out at a potential window of +0.9 V to -0.2 V at a scan rate of 0.05 Vs^{-1}. The CV response for different modifications is as follows; a. bare electrode exhibited a cyclic voltammogram with definite oxidation and reduction peaks. The pre-concentration of *E. coli* on the bare electrode exhibits a drop in redox peak current due to the insulating nature of bacterial cells. b. After drop-casting agarose over the working electrode surface (Agr@SPCE), the magnitude of oxidation and reduction peaks decreased further. This showed the diffusion of the redox mediator was thwarted towards the

116

electrode surface. The bacterial pre-concentration results in further dip in the peak current values. c. The final modification includes the drop-casting of CCD and agarose mix over the surface of the working electrode. The notable decline in oxidation and reduction of peak current values was evident. This could be due to the electrostatic repulsion experienced between the negatively charged CCD and $[Fe(CN)_6]^{3-}$ and hence block the electron transfer on the electrode surface (Fig. 6.8A) [482]. Furthermore, the pre-concentrations with a bacterial solution exhibited the lowest peak current values. This is due to the plenty of bacterial cells attached to Agr/CCD@SPCE. The exposed polycationic colistin moiety on the carbon dots selectively binds with a large number of *E. coli* cells resulting in negligible redox peak current.

EIS was also performed to study the electron transfer behaviour of the modified electrodes at each step, and the results are presented as Nyquist plots (Fig. 6.8B). A significant change in R_{ct} values was observed at every modification step. a) The R_{ct} value of the bare electrode was low (21700 Ω) due to the facile electron transfer across the electrode-electrolyte interface. The pre-concentration of bare SPCE with *E. coli* cells resulted in a subdued electron transfer. Hence, the Rct value increased, b) the Agr@SPCE electrode offered higher resistance in electron transfer (Rct ~ 26100), due to which the faradic current reduced. R_{ct} value increased and c) on immobilizing CCD using agarose matrix of agarose polymer due to which the electron transfer was obstructed and hence, the R_{ct} value increases further (as per the mechanism explained in CV). A remarkable increase in charge transfer resistance from 29500 to 1,32,000 Ω was observed after the pre-concentration of bacterial cells on the Agr/CCD@SPCE. This is attributed to the binding of a substantial number of *E. coli* cells with the polycationic colistin moiety of CCD intercalated in an agarose scaffold.

6.2.6.3 Morphological characterization of Agr/CCD@SPCE

The modified SPCE was sequentially characterized by FESEM and non-contact mode AFM to analyze the morphological changes. FESEM imaging was carried out at 30 K magnifications to achieved sharp images with a clear resolution of the bare electrode and agarose coated electrodes (Agr@SPCE) and Agr/CCD@SPCE (as shown in Fig. 6.9A, B & C).

117

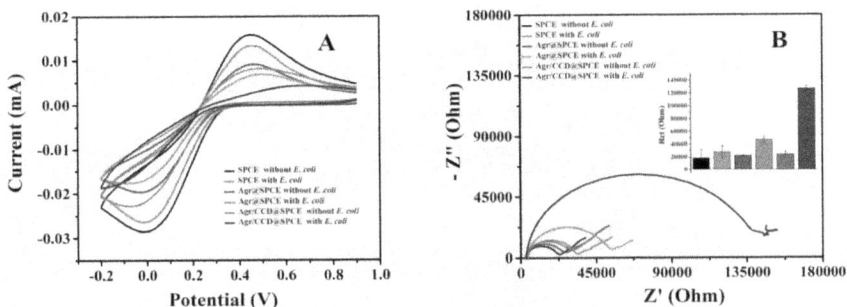

Fig.6.8 Electrochemical response obtained at the different stages of sensor fabrication with and without the presence of E. coli (A) cyclic voltammogram and (B) Nyquist plot

The samples were gold-sputtered before SEM imaging. To begin with, the bare electrode was imaged, and the irregular granular graphitic particles of size ~50 nm were dispersed throughout. The elemental mapping showed the presence of carbon only (Fig. 6.10A) which was obvious because of the carbon printed electrodes. The Agr@SPCE was imaged at a similar magnification, and a uniform coating was observed having a smooth surface with no irregularities. The elemental mapping projects the presence of carbon and oxygen only with different colours, as displayed in Fig. 6.10B. The final modification i.e., Agr/CCD@SPCE, was imaged under similar image acquisition parameters. The difference between agarose and agarose coated CCD was not clearly evident due to the imaging restrictions of the minute size of CCD using SEM. Therefore, the presence of CCD within the agarose matrix was verified by elemental mapping. This was achieved by projecting elements such as carbon, oxygen and nitrogen with different colours, as shown in Fig. 6.10C.

The SEM images of bare SPCE electrode, Agr@SPCE and Agr/CCD@SPCE in the presence of *E. coli* is demonstrated in Fig. 6.9D, E & F. The SEM image of bare electrode did not show any affinity towards *E. coli,* and hence none of the cells were attached on the surface (Fig. 6.9D). The Agr@SPCE shown a few *E. coli* cells embedded into the agarose scaffold/ matrix. The property of agarose dried films to swell in the presence of liquid solvent may allow a smaller number of *E. coli* cells to hold on the surface of the electrode, as shown in Fig. 6.9E. The Agr/CCD@SPCE has shown a greater affinity towards *E. coli* cells due to the presence of colistin-modified CD. The higher number of *E. coli* cells are attached on the modified electrode surface

118

as shown in Fig. 6.9F, and therefore, the higher impedance response was obtained during electrochemical characterization of Agr/CCD@SPCE.

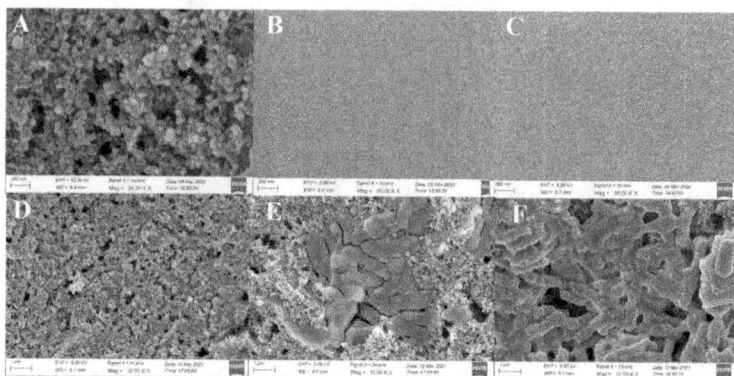

Fig.6.9. Systematic morphological characterization using FESEM image acquisition of (A, D) Bare electrode in absence and presence of E. coli, (B, E) Agr@SPCE in absence and presence of E. coli and (C, F) Agr/CCD@SPCE in absence and presence of E. coli

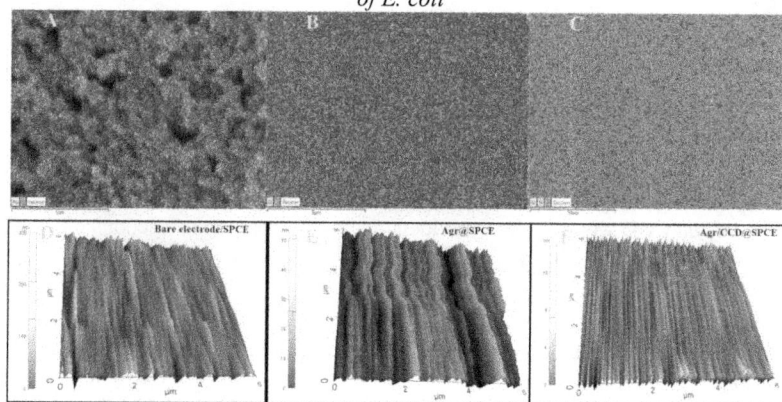

Fig. 6.10 Elemental mapping of A) bare electrode, B) Agr@SPCE, and C) Agr/CCD@SPCE to confirm the immobilization of CCD within agarose scaffold. AFM images of bare electrode D), Agr@SPCE E), and Agr/CCD@SPCE F)

The morphological characterization of Agr/CCD@SPCE was also carried out by AFM to analyze the surface topography and roughness. The AFM images of the bare electrode, agarose coated SPCE, and Agr/CCD@SPCE were snapped at a scan rate of 0.5 Hz with the scan area of 6μ X 6μ (as shown in Fig. 6.10D, E & F). Post imaging, the processed images were analyzed using AFM software to realize the variation in roughness quotient in each modification. It has been observed that the roughness quotient was decreasing from the bare electrode to agarose coated SPCE to Agr/CCD@SPCE. The substantial dip in roughness value from the bare electrode to agarose coated SPCE is because of the polymer coating. The vacant spaces of the agarose matrix are filled by CCD after introducing carbon dots within the polymer scaffold. This perhaps resulted in further reduction of roughness value and confirmed the presence of CCD within agarose dried films.

The SEM images of *E. coli* and *S. aureus* binding to the surface of Agr/CCD@SPCE has been shown in Fig. 6.11. The images clearly demonstrate the higher affinity of the modified electrodes towards *E. coli* as compare to *S. aureus*.

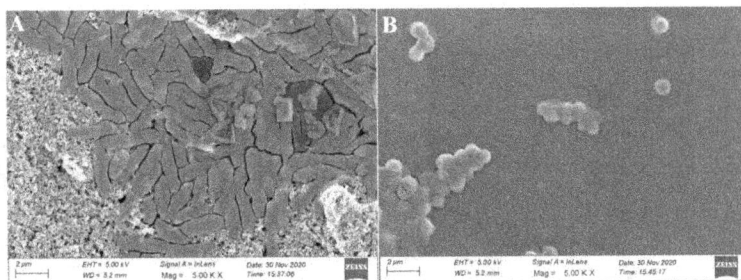

Fig. 6.11 SEM images of Agr/CCD@SPCE with E. coli (A) and S. aureus (B)

6.2.7 Quantitative detection of *E. coli* using Agr/CCD@SPCE sensor

The analytical detection of *E. coli* was performed using Agr/CCD@SPCE in a standardized experimental set-up. The samples with different *E. coli* concentrations (10^2 - 10^8 CFU mL^{-1}) were prepared by serial dilution of the stock culture using 0.1 M PBS and pre-concentrated on the modified Agr/CCD@SPCE electrode. After pre-concentration, the R_{ct} values were measured using EIS. Fig. 6.12 represents the linear increase in the impedance with the bacterial concentration ranges from 10^2 - 10^8 CFU mL^{-1}. The linear increase in impedance can be attributed to the hindrance in electron transfer across the electrode-electrolyte interface offered by the bacteria attached to the electrode surface. The bacteria cells were quantified using Agr/CCD@SPCE in triplicates to ensure the repeatability of the optimized system. The inset in Fig. 6.12 shows the R_{ct} values versus logarithmic concentration of *E. coli* cells (10^2 - 10^8 CFU mL^{-1}) and exhibited a linear relationship. The equation of linear regression is as follows: $R_{ct} = 14085$ CFU mL^{-1} +12951.26 and R-square value = 0.98. The detection limit (S/N = 3) of Agr/CCD@SPCE was calculated as 1.57 CFU mL^{-1}, and the quantification limit was 10^2 CFU mL^{-1} with a pre-concentration step.

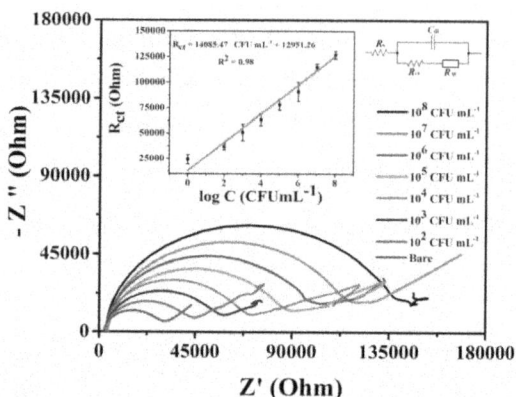

Fig. 6.12 Nyquist plot of Agr/CCD@SPCE in the presence of various E. coli concentrations ranges from $10^2 - 10^8$ CFU mL^{-1}, (inset) linear plot based on the triplicate measurement and equivalent circuit model used for the data analysis

6.2.8 Selectivity of Agr/CCD@SPCE towards *E. coli* in a polymicrobial solution

The selectivity of the Agr/CCD@SPCE was screened in two phases *i)* The EIS response of the sensor electrode to different micro-organisms (*Escherichia coli, Staphylococcus aureus, Proteus vulgaris* and *Mycobacterium smegmatis*) were measured separately in triplicates (Fig.6.13A). The bacterial concentration for all four microbes was fixed at 10^8 CFU mL^{-1}. The measured EIS exhibits a higher response for *E. coli* in comparison to other microbes. As discussed above, the higher R_{ct} values for *E. coli* were attributed to the large number of bacteria attached to the electrode surface. The low R_{ct} values for *S. aureus* and *M. smegmatis* can be explained based on the subdued interaction between colistin moiety of CCD and Gram-positive bacteria due to the absence of LPS membrane. Surprisingly, the R_{ct} values for *P. vulgaris* were much lower than a typical response from Gram-negative bacteria (as in *E. coli*). This is because the *P. vulgaris* exhibited natural resistance against colistin [483,484] and hence, the lower interaction displayed between colistin and *P. vulgaris*.

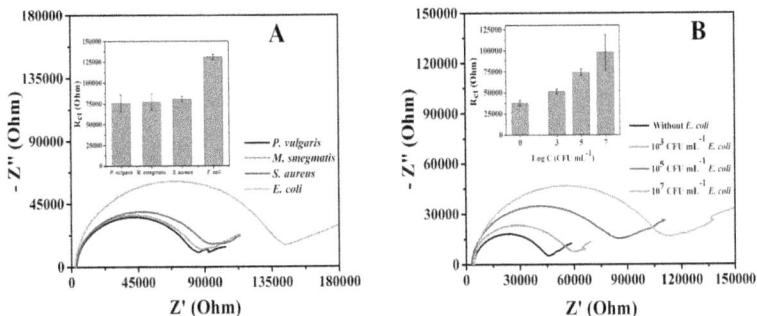

Fig.6.13. The selectivity of Agr/CCD@SPCE - EIS response of (A) different micro-organisms at 10^8 CFU mL^{-1} bacterial concentration (inset: histogram of Agr/CCD@SPCE response for different bacteria) and (B) polymicrobial mixture of all the four micro-organisms with only the concentration of E. coli varying from zero to 10^7 CFU mL^{-1} (inset: histogram of Agr/CCD@SPCE response for different concentration of E. coli in polymicrobial solution)

The impedance measurements were carried out in a polymicrobial mixture of all four micro-organisms. The polymicrobial mixture was prepared by using a varying concentration of E. coli from zero to 10^7 CFU mL^{-1} while keeping the concentration of all the other microbes as 10^5 CFU mL^{-1}. The R_{ct} of the Agr/CCD@SPCE was changing according to the change in E.coli concentrations as displayed in Fig.6.13B. This is due to the selective nature of the developed sensor towards E.coli provided by the colistin moiety of CCD.

6.2.9 Storage stability of Agr/CCD@SPCE

The shelf life of Agr/CCD@SPCE sensors has been monitored over a period of 32 days, as shown in Fig. 6.14. The electrodes were fabricated under similar conditions and stored at room temperature, and impedance measurements were carried out at a regular interval of 8 days. The experiment was performed to measure the repeatable impedimetric response of Agr/CCD@SPCE. The impedimetric response of the developed electrode was estimated using freshly prepared E. coli cells (10^5 CFU mL^{-1}). The measured response was found to be precise and stable when tested on days 1, 8, 16, 24 & 32. This study indicates the potential long-term stability of Agr/CCD@SPCE without any special requirement for the storage of the electrodes. We believe that the sensor can be stored even for a longer duration at room temperature without any special storage condition.

122

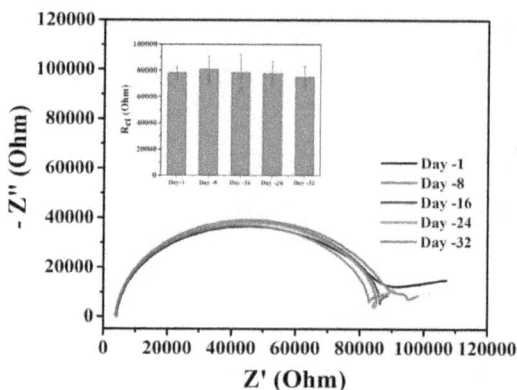

Fig. 6.14 Stability assessment of Agr/CCD@SPCE by measuring the response of the sensor from different modified electrodes stored for a different time period

6.2.10 Detection of *E. coli* in real samples

Table 6.1 shows the percentage recovery of different concentrations of *E. coli* spiked tap water and urine samples obtained using Agr/CCD@SPCE. All the analyses with different concentrations of *E. coli* exhibited excellent recovery. We found a higher percentage recovery in tap water samples compared to that of urine samples. Various ions and minerals present in tap water and urine did not influence the quantification of *E. coli*. This indicates the sensitivity, specificity, and efficiency of the fabricated sensor for detecting *E. coli* in various real samples.

Table 6.1 Percentage recovery estimation of E. coli cells in tap water and urine

Sample	Spiked concentration (CFU mL⁻¹)	Measured concentration (CFU mL⁻¹)	Recovery (%)
	8	7.84	98.0
Tap water	5	4.62	92.4
	3	2.75	91.6
	8	6.73	84.1
Urine	5	4.83	96.6
	3	2.72	90.6

6.2.11 Comparison of the sensor performance

The performance characteristics such as the linear range of detection, lowest detection limit, and electrochemical techniques used for the analysis of the present work compared with those reported in the literature are given in Table 6.2.

Table 6.2. Comparative analysis of the performance characteristics of Agr/CCD@SPCE with the reported polymer based impedimetric sensors for the detection of bacteria

S. No.	Electrode material	Electrochemical technique used	Detection range (CFU mL⁻¹)	LOD/Q (CFU mL⁻¹)	Ref.
1	MIL-53(Fe)/PEDOT composite	EIS , DPV	$2.1 \times 10^2 - 10^8$	4	[485]
2	Polyaniline (PANI) film	EIS	$10^2 - 10^7$	-	[486]
3	3D Ag Nano flower	EIS	$3.0 \times 10^2 - 10^8$	100	[487]
4	Gold nanoparticles-graphene	EIS	$1.5 \times 10^3 - 10^7$	1.5×10^3	[488]
5	bi-functional glucose oxidase-polydopamine nanocomposites and Prussian blue	CV, Amperometric	$10^2 - 10^6$	10^2	[489]
6	Bacteria-imprinted polypyrrole (BIP) film	EIS	$10^3 - 10^8$	10^3	[490]
7	Poly [pyrrole-co-3-carboxyl-pyrrole] copolymer and aptamer	EIS	$10^2 - 10^8$	3	[491]
8	Poly(3-hexylthiophene)-b-poly(3-triethylene-glycol-thiophene)(P3HT-b-P3TEGT)	EIS	$10^3 - 10^7$	500	[274]
9	Agr/CCD@SPCE	EIS	$10^2 - 10^8$	1.575	This work

Despite being such a promising outcome exhibited by Agr/CCD@SPCE, a few limitations cannot be ignored. The fabrication of Agr/CCD@SPCE includes manual drop-casting resulting in inevitable minor variations in the uniformity and diameter of dried agarose films.

This could be overcome by introducing automation in drop-casting for achieving the uniformity of dried agarose films. The behaviour of the developed sensors has been screened in a few real samples, such as tap water and human urine, but the impedance response might vary in a different biological matrix. The measurement of impedance response needs to be done with other clinical samples such as blood, saliva, and sweat on a large scale for calibrating the developed impedimetric sensor.

6.3 Conclusion

The presented work describes the feasibility of colistin functionalized carbon dots immobilized agarose dried films on SPCE (Agr/CCD@SPCE) to fabricate impedimetric sensors for the ultrasensitive detection of *E. coli* bacteria. The electrochemical and microscopic characterization of Agr/CCD@SPCE affirms the immobilization of CCD on SPCE. The impedimetric response of Agr/CCD@SPCE in the presence and absence of *E. coli* suggest the sensitive approach of the developed sensor. The morphological studies were carried out using SEM, and the results complemented the electrochemical characterization of Agr/CCD@SPCE. The quantification of *E. coli* cells was achieved for a broad range from 10^2 to 10^8 CFU mL^{-1} with a detection limit of 1.57 CFU mL^{-1}. The selectivity of the developed sensor was screened in polymicrobial solution and was found to be highly specific to *E. coli* cells. The shelf life of Agr/CCD@SPCE was also tested for 32 days, and the response of the sensor was constant throughout the storage span for a particular concentration of *E. coli* cells. This suggests the stability of the developed sensor is excellent and can be used for a significant time invariably. Agr/CCD@SPCE also exhibited a remarkable percentage recovery for different concentrations of *E. coli* in the case of real samples such as tap water and urine.

Chapter 7

Conclusion and Future Scope

7. Conclusion and future scope

7.1 Conclusion

Fluorimetric and impedimetric sensors have been successfully designed based on surface functionalized carbon dots for bio-imaging and selective identification of pathogenic bacteria. The fluorimetric sensors work on the principle of fluorescence emission obtained from the carbon dots tagged bacterial cells. On the other hand, the impedimetric sensors work on the principle of charge transfer resistance measurement at the electrode-electrolyte interface to specifically detect Gram-negative bacteria.

Carbon dots based fluorimetric sensors was developed for imaging different pathogenic bacteria such as *Escherichia coli*, *Staphylococcus aurues*, *Pseudomonas aeurginosa*, *Bacillus subtilis*, *Proteus vulgaris* and *Klebsiella pneumoniae*. The first variant of carbon dots (NSCD) was synthesized using novel combination of thiourea and 50X TAE buffer to obtain nitrogen and sulphur co-doped carbon dots. The spectral properties of NSCD suggested the bulk fluorescence emission due to the presence of various surface functionalities. The non-toxic nature of NSCD was investigated and it was found to be compatible with bacterial cells with over 96% cell viability even after 24 hours of incubation. The synthesized NSCD was used for bacterial cell tagging analysis with significant fluorescence emission from bacteria. The multi-emissive nature of NSCD was also screened with the tagged *E. coli* cells at different excitation filters such as UV (350-380 nm), blue (415-450 nm) and green (470-525 nm) exhibiting corresponding emission colours such as blue, green and red. Another variant (Cy@CD) of nitrogen and sulphur co-doped carbon dots was synthesized in a similar manner using Cysteamine and 50X TAE precursors. The spectral properties of heteroatomic doped Cy@CD exhibited brilliant fluorescence emission at multiple excitations. The synthesized NSCD probes have excellent photo-stability and biocompatibility providing a facile method for bacterial cell imaging with multi-colour emission that can be extended to image multiple bacteria effectively.

To further achieve an easy method for bacterial cell imaging, a unique pH-sensitive nitrogen doped carbon dots (NtCD) was synthesized using citric acid and glycine. The PL emission was tested at varying pH (1 to 11) with a strong and stable

PL intensity at observed at pH 2 along with high quantum yield (27.2%). The pathogenic bacteria such as *E. coli* and *S. aureus* were tagged with NtCD at various pH (2-9). It was found that the best `tagging pH' was pH 2. The zeta potential analysis explains that the electrostatic interaction between NtCD and pathogenic bacteria facilitated the cell tagging assay. The unique multicolor emissive property was also observed from NtCD tagged pathogenic bacteria.

The fluorimetric method for selective identification of Gram-negative bacteria was developed using colistin antibiotic as a surface passivating agent in the microwave-assisted synthesis of multi-emissive carbon dots (m-CCD). The affinity of m-CCD was found to be higher for Gram-negative bacteria. The selective binding property of the m-CCD was utilized for the quantification of *E. coli* present in various samples such as standard sample, tap water and human urine with broad detection range and good linearity.

The selective nature of m-CCD was explored intuitively by the tagging of Gram-negative over Gram-positive bacteria. The fluorescence imaging of m-CCD tagged Gram-negative bacteria such as *E. coli* and *P. aeruginosa* exhibited strong fluorescence. The m-CCD did not show tagging with Gram-positive bacteria such as *S. aureus* and *B. subtilis* resulting in no fluorescence at all excitation wavelengths. Finally, the selectivity of m-CCD was also confirmed by detecting *E. coli* cells in a polymicrobial sample.

A single-step facile hydrothermal synthesis of colistin passivated carbon dots (CCD) was achieved using citric acid, ethylenediamine, and colistin precursors. The CCD was used for the fabrication of label-free, disposable impedimetric sensor for the detection of *E. coli* by immobilizing it on screen-printed carbon electrodes in an agarose matrix (Agr/CCD@SPCE). The impedimetric sensor was thoroughly characterized and tested with samples containing *E.coli* using electroanalytical techniques. EIS analysis was carried out with a wide range of bacterial concentrations (10^2 - 10^8 CFU mL^{-1}) and found that the charge transfer resistance was linearly increasing with bacterial concentration. The specificity of Agr/CCD@SPCE was tested for various bacterial strains and it was found to be selective to *E. coli*. The selectivity of Agr/CCD@SPCE was further evaluated by testing it with polymicrobial samples containing *S. aureus*, *P. vulgaris* and *M. smegmatis* with varying

127

concentrations of *E. coli*. The sensor performance was also tested with real samples such as tap water and human urine and it exhibited a sensitive response towards different concentrations of *E. coli*. In addition, several electrodes were fabricated under similar conditions and stored at room temperature to evaluate the shelf life of Agr/CCD@SPCE. EIS measurements were carried out at a regular interval of eight days in a solution containing *E. coli* cells and obtained a precise and stable response for the entire duration.

Therefore, sensitive and selective detection of multiple pathogenic bacteria was achieved by fluorimetric and impedimetric methods using novel carbon dots. The developed sensors exhibited excellent detection range with high selectivity for specific bacterial cells in polymicrobial samples. The fluorimetric and impedimetric-based bacterial detection possess a holistic approach in the clinical investigation to identify several pathogens on a single platform to achieve a rapid, portable, and cost-effective diagnostic setup.

7.2 Future Scope

In this thesis, we have discussed the development of fluorimetric and impedimetric sensors for the detection of multiple pathogenic bacteria causing lethal diseases such as sepsis, tuberculosis, cholera, urinary tract infection, MRSA infection, syphilis, gonorrhea and respiratory tract related diseases.

The developed heteroatomic doped fluorogenic carbon dots for multicolour bacterial cell imaging application was tested in standard sample. This can be extented to test samples with different matrix such as real samples (drinking water, fruit juices) and clinical samples (blood/ serum, urine and saliva). Hence, synthesis of fluorogenic carbon dots based sensors for imaging bacterial cells in biological samples will form an inherent part of our future works.

A highly selective fluorimetric sensor based on colistin modified carbon dots was developed to recognize and quantify Gram-negative bacteria. The carbon dots can be modified with different antibiotics such as vancomycin and quaternary ammonium compounds to make it specific for the detection of Gram-positive bacteria. Similarly, the fluorimetric sensors can also be redesign by using different surface passivating agents for the specific detection of different pathogenic bacteria.

A label-free impedimetric sensor was developed by immobilizing agarose mixed colistin carbon dots on the surface of SPCE for the specific detection of *E. coli* cells. The polymer agarose can be replaced with potential polymers such as polyvinyl alcohol (PVA) and conducting polymers like polyaniline mixed with surface passivated carbon dots for the selective detection of pathogenic bacteria with enhanced sensitivity. Moreover, the lyophilized carbon dots can also be mixed with conducting ink and used for the fabricatoin of electrode with higher selectivity and sensitivity.

The presented fluorimetric and impedimetric sensors for the detection of pathogenic bacteria can only be used in laboratory settings. To upscale the feasibilty of the sensors for the end-user usage, these sensors can be integrated with lab-on-chip devices to develop POCT devicse for the detection of multiple pathogenic bacteria with high throughput and utmost commercial viability.

www.ingramcontent.com/pod-product-compliance
Lightning Source LLC
Chambersburg PA
CBHW071424210326
41597CB00020B/3643